The Power of Bedside Manners in Patient Care

The Power of Bedside Manners in Patient Care: A Timeless Prescription

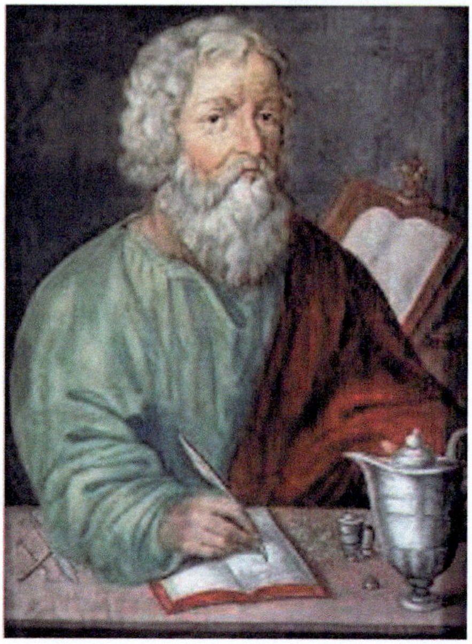

Portrait of Hippocrates (1787), by the Majorat of Setúbal.

Seems to have been based on this 1584 line engraving of Hippocrates (Wellcome Collection).

A Guide for Healthcare Providers to Learn the Art of Medicine

Barry Silverman

The Power of Bedside Manners in Patient Care

A Healthcare Provider's Guide

Springer

Barry Silverman
Medicine
Emory University
Brookhaven, GA, USA

ISBN 978-3-032-10495-3 ISBN 978-3-032-10496-0 (eBook)
https://doi.org/10.1007/978-3-032-10496-0

This Springer imprint is published by the registered company Springer Nature Switzerland AG
The registered company address is: Gewerbestrasse 11, 6330 Cham, Switzerland

Preface

Healing Bedside Manners

He walks the halls with quiet grace,
A steady calm upon his face.
Not rushed, not distant, never cold—
But present, warm, and gently bold.

He knows the science, charts, and scans,
The medicine that steadies hands.
But more than that, he reads the eyes,
The unsaid fears, the stifled cries.

He pulls a chair, not just a chart,
And listens first, with open heart.
Each word he speaks, both kind and clear,
Makes pain feel seen and hope draw near.

He doesn't talk at—he speaks with—
A gift too rare, a healing myth.
And in that space, the patient finds
Their dignity, their peace of mind.

He sees not cases, beds, or files,
But lives and souls and trembling trials.
He holds their stories, grief, and grace,
And never once looks through a face.

So trust walks in when he appears,
And silence yields to shared frontiers.
For healing starts not just in blood,
But in the quiet, human flood—
Of voice, of care, of gentle art:
A doctor skilled in healing hearts.

Medicine is both an art and a science. While **classrooms and clinics** train future physicians in diagnosis and treatment, something crucial is often overlooked: the deeply human act of truly caring for another person.

Across cultures and centuries, legendary physicians like Hippocrates, Paracelsus, Francis Peabody, and William Osler have championed this idea—reminding us that

compassion, respect, and trust are as vital as scientific knowledge. Hippocrates declared, *Wherever the art of medicine is loved, there is also love of humanity.* Paracelsus argued that doctors must understand not just symptoms, but the whole person. He said, *Medicine is not only a science; It is also an art. It does not consist of compounding pills and plasters; it deals with the very processes of life. Which must be understood before they may be guided.* Frances Peabody observed, *One of the essential qualities of the clinician is interest in humanity, for the secret of the care of the patient is in caring for the patient.* Osler urged his students to look beyond disease and see the patient's full humanity. Yet, in modern medical training, these timeless lessons are too often encountered only by chance—passed down through an inconsistent "hidden curriculum." As a result, empathy and authentic connection are now endangered skills.

There is a link between how doctors communicate with patients and the trust and confidence that patients have in their physician [1]. Research has shown that how physicians communicate with their patients, and how they make them feel, have a large impact on whether doctors face malpractice lawsuits [2]. A good bedside manner is far more effective in reducing the risk of medical malpractice. This was pointed out in an article called defensive medicine in the *New York Times*. Patients who placed the most malpractice lawsuits were those that felt their doctors ignored them, rushed them, or failed to explain things adequately.

A Missing Curriculum

Despite a rich legacy, formal instruction in the art of medicine is rare. Students master anatomy, pathophysiology, and pharmacology—but the artful skills of *communication, compassion, and connection* are relegated to informal learning, risking missed opportunities and perpetuating old habits.

The Vital Role of Communication

Doctor-patient communication is foundational. Every encounter unfolds between unequal partners, often under emotional, stressful, or vulnerable circumstances—and complicated by differences in gender, culture, age, and more. Patients seek two things: to know and understand, and to feel known and understood.

However, studies show communication skills often decline as training progresses. Many physicians avoid discussing emotional or social issues, citing lack of time or a belief that they can't help managing these concerns. Yet evidence shows that taking the time to listen and understand improves efficiency, patient satisfaction, and outcomes. Effective communication means learning the patient's story: their daily life, their relationships, their worries, beliefs, work pressures, and expectations. It is about listening—not just talking—to develop genuine trust.

Osler summarized his approach with two Greek words: **Philotechnia** ("love of the art") and **Philantropia** ("love of humanity"). The ideal physician combines technical skill with moral sensitivity, trustworthiness, and a willingness to invest in each patient's well-being.

Why It Matters

A communication gap in medicine is more than frustrating—it is harmful. Patients crave genuine connection: reassurance, understanding, and acknowledgment, not just diagnoses and prescriptions. Families, too, suffer without open dialogue. As Dr. Melvin Casberg observed, "the art of medicine disappears with each practitioner and must be learned anew by every generation." This book is my attempt to fill that void—to give students and clinicians a practical guide for compassionate, high-quality care.

What Every Student Should Master

The **art of medicine** must be taught intentionally and consistently. Here are the core elements every student should embrace:

- **Deep Listening**—Hearing the patient's whole story without interruption.
- **Seeing the Whole Person**—Recognizing the patient's identity, values, daily life, and support systems.
- **Skillful Touch**—Bringing presence and respect to the physical exam.
- **Empathy in Action**—Feeling *with* the patient, not just feeling *for* them.
- **Earning Trust**—Building relationships through integrity, transparency, and consistency.
- **Courage and Accountability**—Owning mistakes and advocating for patients.
- **Connecting with Families**—Engaging loved ones with respect and inclusivity.
- **Civility in Practice**—Treating every member of the healthcare team with dignity.

These are not luxuries. They are therapeutic interventions in their own right.

Manners-Based Medicine

During my time teaching at Grady Memorial Hospital, I often see talented clinicians who struggle to connect beyond medical facts. Patients frequently tell me no doctor has asked about their lives, joys, or hardships. We must **revive the art of conversation**—what I call "Manners-Based Medicine." Just as science grounds evidence-based medicine, manners-based medicine grounds care in human respect and connection.

Reviving Mentorship

The most meaningful lessons in medicine often come from mentors—not textbooks. It is critical that today's role models exemplify communication, empathy, and clinical excellence. Seek mentors who lead not just with words, but through everyday example—embodying integrity, skill, and inclusion.

The Joy of Practicing the Art

As Dr. Philip Tumulty once said, *good medicine brings the thrill of bringing relief to fellow human beings and the daily experience of seeing and understanding more clearly the depths of human nature. The clinician is not a detached observer, but an engaged participant in the human experience.* **This is the true art of medicine:** a practice where science and humanity meet, and each patient encounter is an opportunity to heal, connect, and uplift.

Brookhaven, GA, USA Barry Silverman

References

1. Ha JF, Longneker N. Doctor-patient communication: a review. Ochsner J. 2010;10:38–43
2. Jena AB, Seabury S, Lakawalla D, Chandra A. Malpractice risk according to physician specialty. NEJM. 2011; 365:629–36. https://doi.org/10.1056/NEJMsa1012370

Contents

The Mastery of Bedside Manners: Essential to the Practice of Medicine

1

The Importance of Bedside Manner in Medicine

In the practice of medicine, the healthcare provider's scientific knowledge and technical expertise are undeniably critical to patient care, but it is equally important to recognize the value of bedside manners. Bedside manners are the way you communicate with and attend to patients, encompassing not only verbal communication but also non-verbal cues, empathy, and overall attitude. The significance of good bedside manners lies not just in fostering a compassionate doctor-patient relationship but also in promoting better clinical outcomes, enhancing patient satisfaction, and supporting the holistic well-being of the individual receiving care [2] (Fig. 1.1).

B. Silverman, *The Power of Bedside Manners in Patient Care*,
https://doi.org/10.1007/978-3-032-10496-0_1

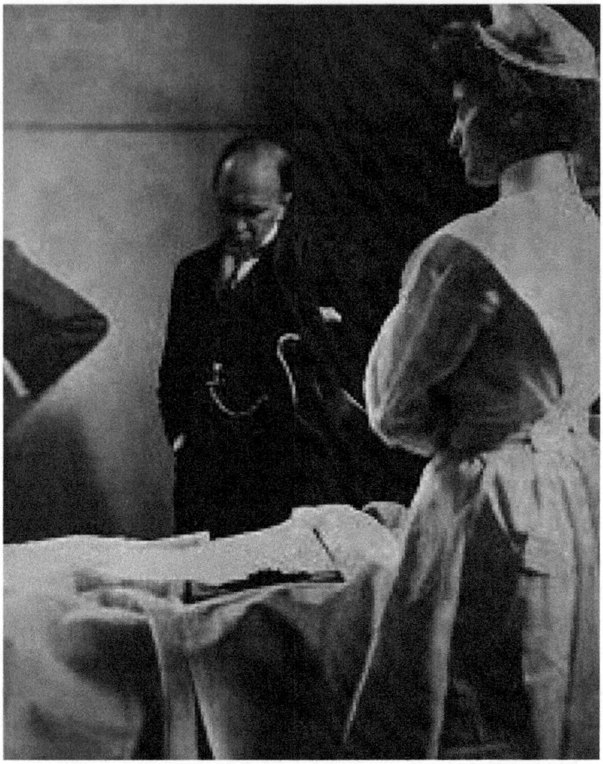

Fig. 1.1 Sir William Osler (1849–1919), reading a patient's chart at bedside as a nurse watches. Osler was the first professor of medicine at John Hopkins University Medical School. (Photo courtesy of Mark Silverman estate)The writing and teaching of William Osler set the standard for humanism, science, and patient care in medicine. The book The Quotable Osler by William Osler ed by Mark Silverman, J Jock Murray, and Charles Bryan is a treasure house of advice on bedside manners [1]

The Role of Bedside Manner in Patient Care

At its core, bedside manner involves empathy, respect, and attentiveness. Patients are often in vulnerable states, dealing with illness, uncertainty, and fear. The health-care provider who demonstrates genuine concern, actively listens to the patient's concerns, and explains the diagnosis and treatment options in clear, understandable language can help alleviate anxiety and build trust. Good bedside manner can transform a routine medical encounter into a positive experience, contributing to the patient's emotional and psychological comfort. This is crucial, as patients who feel heard and respected are more likely to adhere to medical advice and follow prescribed treatments [3].

A key aspect of bedside manner is communication. A healthcare provider with strong communication skills can break down complex medical information into terms the patient can understand, ensuring that the patient feels informed and empowered to make decisions about their own care. Clear communication also extends to addressing concerns and answering questions, no matter how insignificant they may seem. When patients feel their concerns are taken seriously, they are more likely to engage in their treatment plan actively and cooperatively.

The Psychological Impact of a Healthcare Provider's Attitude

The psychological impact of your demeanor should not be underestimated. Studies have shown that patients who perceive their healthcare providers as compassionate and attentive tend to have lower levels of stress and anxiety [4, 5] This in turn can improve overall health outcomes, Words matter, attentive listening is essential, a cold, detached, or rushed approach will make patients feel neglected or dismissed, potentially leading to feelings of alienation or fear. When you are dismissive of a patient's symptoms or fail to provide clear explanations, it can lead to frustration, confusion, or even a reluctance to seek care in the future. However, if you are, compassionate and use a patient-centered approach this will foster collaboration and strengthen the doctor-patient relationship, which is vital for successful treatment.

Physical cues—such as making eye contact, using a calm tone of voice, and sitting at the patient's level—contribute significantly to how a patient feels during an interaction. Small gestures like a reassuring touch or an attentive listening posture convey a sense of care and attentiveness. These non-verbal cues complement the verbal communication and help in building rapport, reinforcing the message that the doctor sees the patient as a person rather than just a case to be treated.

The Impact on Medical Outcomes

Although bedside manner may seem like a soft skill in comparison to technical knowledge, its effects can directly influence medical outcomes. Research has shown that patients who have positive interactions with their doctors are more likely to adhere to prescribed treatment regimens, attend follow-up appointments, and trust their physician's advice [6]. This compliance can lead to better management of chronic conditions, faster recovery from illnesses, and a lower likelihood of medical errors. Additionally, when doctors make the effort to engage with patients in a meaningful way, they are often able to gather more comprehensive medical histories and catch potential complications that might otherwise go unnoticed.

The relationship between bedside manner and medical outcomes is not confined to patient satisfaction alone. There is evidence suggesting that doctors with strong communication skills may experience fewer malpractice claims [7] This is because the perception of good communication and empathy helps prevent misunderstandings and cultivates a sense of partnership between doctor and patient, reducing the likelihood of disputes or dissatisfaction with care.

Challenges in Modern Medicine

Despite its importance, practicing good bedside manner is not always easy. The modern healthcare environment, particularly in hospitals and busy medical practices, often places immense pressure on healthcare providers. Time constraints, administrative tasks, and the increasing complexity of patient care can make it difficult for you to dedicate the time and attention necessary to develop meaningful relationships with each patient. Additionally, the stress and demands of practice may cause you to experience burnout, which can impact their ability to provide compassionate care. Nevertheless, many argue that fostering a strong bedside manner is an essential component of preventing burnout as it creates more fulfilling and human-centered interactions within the healthcare system [8].

The Importance of Civility and Courtesy

In an era dominated by cutting-edge technology and revolutionary medical treatments, it may seem unnecessary to emphasize the value of good manners in healthcare. After all, most of us entered the field with a shared mission: to help people, driven by compassion and the desire to alleviate suffering. We learned our social behaviors early on, and as caregivers, we assume that treating others with respect comes naturally. Yet, despite these good intentions, many patients still experience doctors, nurses, and office staff who can come across as dismissive, uncommunicative, or downright rude. The absence of courtesy in medicine isn't just about politeness—it is about respecting the individual.

The Impact of Your Behavior on Patient Outcomes

Are you making eye contact with your patients? Are you really listening when they speak, or are you distracted by a phone call or the screen of an electronic medical record (EMR)? Are you consistently late to appointments? These behaviors may seem minor, but they can have a significant impact on patient satisfaction and, ultimately, on health outcomes. As Austin Flint Sr., a prominent figure in American medicine, once said, *the life of a sick person can be shortened not only by the acts but by the words and manner of the physician. It is, therefore, a sacred duty to guard himself carefully in this respect and to avoid all things which have a tendency to discourage the patient and to depress his spirits.* The simple truth is this: poor manners can undermine trust, breed anxiety, and even compromise treatment. When patients feel disregarded or dismissed, it can affect their willingness to fully engage in their care, follow medical advice, or even return for future appointments.

The Patient as a Persson Is Your First Priority

In healthcare, the patient requires our full attention. Every interruption—whether it's a phone call, a nurse barging in, or the physician focusing more on the EMR than the patient—can disrupt not only the dialogue but also the trust and connection that form the foundation of effective care. Tardiness, with doctors running late or patients waiting for extended periods, is a form of disrespect. When patients feel their time is undervalued, it can have a lasting impact on their experience and trust in the system.

Why Trust Matters in Medicine

Surprisingly, healthcare institutions—where patient satisfaction is paramount—often lag behind other service industries, like hospitality, in terms of courtesy and professionalism. But here's the irony: good manners aren't just "nice to have"—they directly impact patient outcomes. Poor medical outcomes rarely stem from a lack of medical knowledge. Instead, they often arise from poor communication and a lack of rapport between doctor and patient. Trust is crucial in medicine, and it is built on positive interactions. A patient who feels respected and listened to is far less likely to sue for malpractice, while a patient who feels dismissed is more likely to question their doctor's competence.

The Hidden Curriculum: Learning Bedside Manners

For many years, medical students learned the art of bedside manners not through formal training, but by observing their mentors—senior physicians with decades of experience at the bedside. Unfortunately, the "hidden curriculum" that once guided these interactions has become less effective in today's fast-paced, tech-driven healthcare landscape. With more emphasis on data, algorithms, and evidence-based guidelines, the personal relationship between physician and patient is sometimes relegated to a secondary concern. Moreover, physicians today are spending more time interacting with technology than with their patients. The warm, face-to-face conversations that were once central to patient care are often viewed as outdated or unnecessary. But the truth is, a compassionate, engaged consultation is more than a "nice gesture" for patients—it's vital. When patients feel heard and understood, they are more likely to trust their physician, comply with treatment plans, and experience better outcomes.

The Power of Communication in Healthcare

Perhaps one of the most effective ways to improve patient satisfaction—and, by extension, health outcomes—is through communication. Taking the time to explain procedures, answer questions, and provide updates builds trust and fosters a sense of security. Patients need to know when to expect their doctor, who will be involved in their care, and what each step of the process entails. When doctors fail to communicate—whether by being unavailable or not explaining what's happening—patients can feel neglected, anxious, or even alienated. This breakdown in communication can ultimately erode trust, creating a barrier to healing.

The Mayo Clinic, renowned for its patient-centered approach, outlined timeless principles in 1927 that emphasized the importance of good manners in medicine. These principles can guide healthcare professionals in cultivating more effective, compassionate patient relationships.

1. **A call from a patient takes precedence over personal engagements.**
2. **Neglecting the patient means you are in the wrong profession.**
3. **A timely smile can often ease the sting of a bad prognosis.**
4. **Taking a personal interest in each patient benefits both the patient and the physician.**
5. **Every patient deserves respect and the utmost courtesy.**
6. **Even seemingly trivial ailments should be treated with care, as they are significant to the patient.**
7. **Knock before entering a room; always respect privacy.**
8. **Avoid unnecessary interruptions during consultations.**
9. **No patient should leave dissatisfied.**
10. **The ability to form a friendship with patients is a key to success in medicine.**
11. **While it's easy to please an easy patient, there's true satisfaction in pleasing a difficult one.**
12. **Bad manners in medicine reflect a fundamental mistake—a misalignment of vocation and practice.**

These principles offer a simple yet powerful framework for improving physician-patient relationships and remind us that good bedside manners are essential to high-quality care.

Conclusion: Medicine Beyond Diagnosis

Bedside manner is an indispensable part of healthcare that extends beyond simply being kind or polite; it is about forming a deep, empathetic connection with patients and offering them not just medical expertise but also emotional support. Healthcare providers who engage with their patients thoughtfully and respectfully improve not only the quality of the patient experience but also the likelihood of positive health outcomes. While the demands of modern medicine can make it challenging to prioritize bedside manner, the benefits—both for the patient and the physician—are too significant to overlook. A compassionate, attentive approach to patient care is as vital as any medical procedure in achieving the best possible outcomes for those in need of care.

In the end, medicine is not just about diagnosing diseases; it's about understanding the person who is the patient. It's about offering a listening ear, a kind word, and, above all, the dignity that every patient deserves. Good manners are not just a social nicety—they are a vital component of the healing process. When we treat patients with kindness, respect, and empathy, we do more than help them feel better; we build the trust and confidence they need to navigate their healing journey. In a world where healthcare can sometimes feel impersonal and mechanized, the human touch—rooted in good manners—remains one of the most powerful tools we have in caring for the whole person.

References

1. Silverman ME, Murray TJ, Bryan CS. The quotable Osler. Philadelphia: American College of Physicians; 2003.
2. Kaplan SH, Greenfield S, Ware JE. Assessing the effects of physician–patient interactions on the outcome of chronic disease. Med Care. 1989;27(Suppl):S110–27.
3. Ghosh AK, Joshi S, Ghosh A. Effective patient–physician communication—a concise review. J Assoc Physicians India. 2020;68(6):53–7.
4. Gullace G, Peirone L. Communication in medicine: part III: psychological aspects of the doctor–patient relationship. EC Cardiol. 2021;8(7):33–9.
5. Goold SD, Lipkin M Jr. The doctor–patient relationship: challenges, opportunities, and strategies. J Gen Intern Med. 1999;14:529–33.
6. Zolnierek KB, Dimatteo MR. Physician communication and patient adherence to treatment: a meta-analysis. Med Care. 2009;47:826–34. https://doi.org/10.1097/MLR.0b013e31819a5acc.
7. Kusmoto F, Ross J, Wright D, Chazai WA, Anderson RE. Analysis of closed claims among all medicals: importance of communication and other non-clinical contributing factors. Risk Manag Healthc Policy. 2024;17:411–22. https://doi.org/10.2147/RMHP.S403710.
8. Wert K, Donaldson AM, Dinh TA, Montero DP, Parry R, Renew JR, et al. Communication training helps to reduce burnout during COVID-19 pandemic. Health Serv Res Manag Epidemiol. 2023;10:23333928221148079. https://doi.org/10.1177/23333928221148079.

2 Distinguishing Between Manners and Etiquette: The Same Dance But Different Steps

Why Are Manners Critical to Our Care of Patients?

> Edmund Burke, the Irish-English statesman and philosopher, once observed, *Manners are of more importance than laws. Upon them, in a great measure, the laws depend. The law touches us but here and there, and now and then. Manners are what vex or soothe, corrupt or purify, exalt or debase, barbarize or refine us, by a constant, steady, uniform, insensible operation, like that of the air we breathe in. They give their whole form and color to our lives. According to their quality, they aid morals, they supply them, or they totally destroy them.*

In medicine, bedside manners hold even more significance than Burke could have imagined. When a patient walks into a doctor's office, they are not only offering their body for examination—they are placing their trust in the hands of the healthcare provider. Exposing oneself to the vulnerability of medical procedures, often invasive or painful, is an act of courage. This moment of emotional and physical exposure demands empathy, respect, and dignity. Patients don't just want treatment—they want to be treated with kindness and courtesy. A little attention to good manners can significantly shape their experience and, by extension, their healing journey (Fig. 2.1).

B. Silverman, *The Power of Bedside Manners in Patient Care*,
https://doi.org/10.1007/978-3-032-10496-0_2

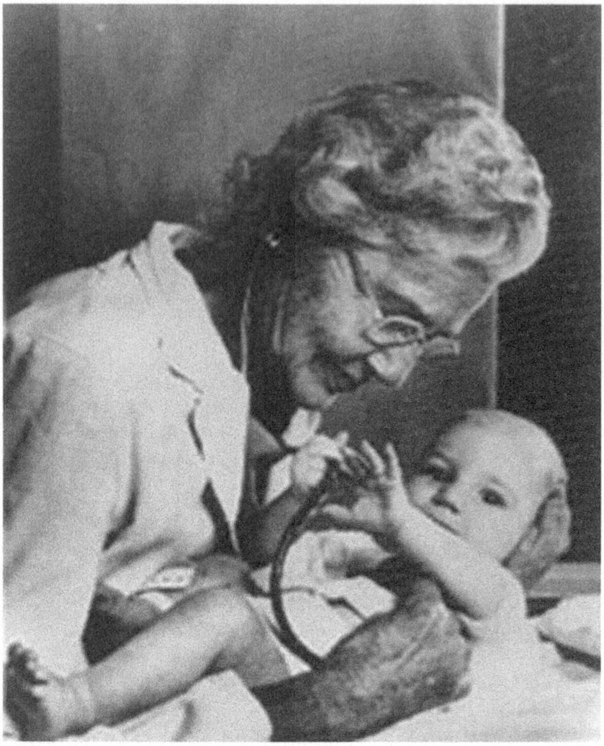

Fig. 2.1 Helen Taussig "Mother of Pediatric Cardiology". (Courtesy of Yousuf Karsh estate)The story of Helen Taussig is about overcoming childhood hardships, systemic, societal, and institutional prejudices, bias, and bigotry. She was a remarkably determined individual who used brilliance, tenacity, patience, and determination to achieve her goals and change medical care. At the bedside and on the ward, she was renowned for her manners and courtesy

Manners vs. Etiquette: What's the Difference?

Manners and etiquette, though often used interchangeably, are not the same. **Manners** are the basic social skills we learn as children—simple acts of politeness like saying "please" and "thank you," or waiting our turn to speak. **Etiquette**, on the other hand, is a more formal set of rules that govern behavior in specific situations, such as how to dine, dress, or interact in professional settings. While traditional etiquette once served as a social code that marked social hierarchies, today, society is more egalitarian, and many see old-fashioned etiquette as unnecessary or even elitist.

However, even in today's more relaxed world, etiquette plays an important role, particularly in professional settings like healthcare. It's not just about saying "hello" or offering a thoughtful gesture—it's about how we present ourselves. In medicine, appearance matters. A neat, well-groomed physician conveys respect for both the patient and the profession. Scruffy, blood-stained scrubs or a disheveled appearance send the opposite message. When you're treated by a doctor who looks polished and professional, you feel more confident in their abilities. The significance of dress and appearance are discussed in detail in Chap. 10.

Rudeness in Society: A Shifting Norm

The cultural shift that began in the 1960s marked a seismic change in how we viewed authority and social conventions. Baby Boomers and members of the Silent Generation rebelled against the formality of previous generations, rejecting established norms and embracing a more informal approach to life. This rebellion didn't just affect fashion; it changed how we interacted with each other. Rudeness, once considered a breach of etiquette, slowly made its way into mainstream culture. Public incivility became common, and a 2002 Pew study revealed that 79% of Americans believed rudeness had become a serious problem, with nearly half admitting to contributing to it [1]. Rudeness has even infiltrated areas once known for decorum—public figures like Donald Trump built careers on shock value, while political discourse often descended into public insults and shouting matches. Society increasingly viewed good manners as quaint and old-fashioned, while rude behavior became a form of entertainment.

Courtesy in Medicine: A Rare Beacon of Respect

Despite this cultural shift, medicine remains a rare beacon of courtesy. In an age where formality and politeness are increasingly dismissed, civility in healthcare continues to be essential. A simple "thank you" is more than just a nicety—it's a recognition of kindness and respect. Active listening, explaining procedures clearly, and treating patients with dignity are not just polite gestures; they are the foundation of effective medical care.

Judith Martin, known as *Miss Manners*, critiques the decline of basic courtesies in healthcare in her book *Miss Manners Rescues Civilization* [2]. She observes the growing disregard for simple acts of respect—patients waiting for hours without explanation, medical staff failing to introduce themselves, and a lack of attention to basic consent before exams. Even the decline in professional attire—doctors showing up in disheveled, overly casual clothing—reflects this shift. While informality may reflect broader societal trends, it can make the patient experience feel impersonal and the care less reassuring.

A New Medical Culture: The Shift Toward Informality

Over the past several decades, medicine has undergone a cultural transformation. After World War II, a wave of returning veterans entered the profession, promoting greater diversity and inclusivity. But it was the social upheaval of the 1960s and 1970s that truly reshaped the medical landscape. Young physicians began to reject the rigid formality that had long defined the profession. The once-mandatory white coat—symbol of authority and detachment—gradually gave way to the more comfortable, accessible look of scrubs, sometimes playfully decorated with colors or cartoons.

This change in attire mirrored a deeper shift in values. Medicine began to favor approachability over hierarchy, and the traditional, top-down doctor-patient relationship started to evolve into a more collaborative partnership. The growing presence of women in medicine accelerated this transformation. Today, women make up more than half of all medical students, challenging outdated gender norms and helping to redefine professional roles. Nurses, once seen as subordinate, are now recognized as critical members of the care team and leaders in clinical decision-making.

Bedside Manners in the Age of Casual Care: A Dying Art?

While informality has brought many positive changes, one essential element has begun to erode: civility. The small but powerful acts that build trust—introducing oneself, explaining procedures, maintaining a professional presence—are too often overlooked. In some hospitals, even the way patients are addressed reflects this shift: referred to not by name, but by room number or diagnosis. Such habits, while perhaps unintentional, can make patients feel invisible and disrespected. Civility in medicine isn't just about politeness—it's about creating a healing space grounded in respect, communication, and trust. Yet many healthcare institutions haven't adjusted to emphasize these values, and the consequences are felt at the bedside.

Learning Bedside Manners

Medical students are typically introduced to the principles of bedside communication early in their training. These lessons stress empathy, attentiveness, and respect. But they're often taught before students have substantial patient contact, and there's an assumption that common courtesy will naturally carry over into clinical care.

While most students begin their training eager to connect with and care for patients, the emotional toll of medicine—grueling hours, constant stress, exposure to suffering—can lead to burnout and emotional withdrawal. As a defense mechanism, some may adopt dark humor or emotional detachment, behaviors that risk appearing cold or indifferent.

Mentorship plays a key role in how students develop their bedside manner. But not all senior physicians model compassionate care. Some, despite their technical brilliance, lack the interpersonal skills that nurture trust. Worse, research reveals that mistreatment of trainees—from verbal abuse to bullying—is still common in medical culture. These negative behaviors can be passed down, learned rather than questioned.

To make matters worse, there's little structured feedback on how students interact with patients. While hospitals may track overall patient satisfaction, medical schools rarely ask patients to evaluate students' bedside behavior. Without meaningful feedback, both positive habits and harmful ones can go unchecked.

Respect: The Cornerstone of Professionalism

Technical knowledge alone does not make a great physician. What sets excellent doctors apart is their ability to communicate clearly, treat others with dignity, and work collaboratively with colleagues. Disrespect—whether toward nurses, patients, or fellow clinicians—can quietly but powerfully sabotage patient care. A brilliant diagnosis means little if the patient feels dismissed or the care team is fractured. As etiquette expert Judith Martin once said, "*A good heart does not automatically translate into good manners*."

The Patient Centered Care: Why Bedside Manners Still Matters

Nowhere is professionalism more visible—or more essential—than at the bedside. The medical encounter breaks many rules of social convention: patients are physically exposed, asked deeply personal questions, and often feel vulnerable. In this delicate context, small gestures matter immensely. Attentive listening, kindness, respect for personal comfort, and a calm, pleasant demeanor can make a lasting impact.

For most patients, medical competence is not judged by degrees or credentials, but by how they're treated as human beings. Bedside manner is the outward expression of inner empathy—conveyed not only by what we say, but by how well we listen and how much we care.

Physician Philip Tumulty captured this truth in a 1970 address to Johns Hopkins medical students:

> *What many patients miss and resent today is the inability to communicate with their physician in a meaningful manner.*
>
> *Patients have questions that need answering, fears that require calming, and misunderstandings that need clarification.*
>
> *Many leave the doctor's office with less understanding of their health than the average car owner has when picking up a repaired vehicle from the garage. And if the patient feels neglected, the family feels completely shut out. No wonder there is resentment.*

What Are We Really Communicating to Patients?

Hospitals and clinics do offer information to patients—but much of it is designed around the convenience of staff, not the needs of patients. Billing procedures, office hours, parking instructions, and hospital rules are often emphasized. What's often missing is meaningful information about the patient's care experience.

Patients are rarely told who will be entering their room, when to expect tests, or how to express personal preferences—such as when not to be disturbed or how they prefer to be addressed. Their rights are often reduced to a brochure or a wall plaque. In practice, it's the patient who is expected to conform to the system—not the system that adjusts to the patient.

What Should We Communicate?

Respect begins with the basics:

- Everyone who interacts with a patient should introduce themselves by name and role.
- Adult patients should be addressed formally by their last name unless invited to do otherwise.
- Before any test or treatment, the patient should be told what it is, why it's being done, and how they'll receive the results.

In the hospital setting, patients should know:

- Who is in charge of their care.
- What treatments or procedures are planned.
- When results will come, and who will explain them.
- What medications they are receiving and why—including potential side effects and expected outcomes.
- When conducting medical rounds, let patients and their families know what time to expect the team.
- Always introduce everyone present, including students and obtain patient permission for the student involvement in teaching rounds.
  Patients have every right to decline participation by unfamiliar staff. At times, hospitalized individuals seem to have fewer recognized rights than those incarcerated.

Why Politeness Still Matters in Modern Medicine

In today's healthcare environment—where collaboration and shared decision-making are the norm—civility is not optional. Every team member, from doctors and nurses to front-desk staff, shapes the patient experience. Disrespect or poor communication can lead to confusion, delay, mistrust, and even medical error. Politeness is not about being superficial—it's about honoring the dignity of every person in the clinical space. Respect builds trust. And trust is the foundation of healing.

References

1. Farkas S, Johnson J. Aggravating circumstances: a status report on rudeness in America. 2002. ISBN 1-889483-75-3.
2. Martin J. Miss manners rescues civilization. New York: Crown Publishers; 1996.

Civility Is a Pillar of Medical Professionalism

3

Civility is a fundamental pillar of the medical profession, essential for fostering trust, ensuring effective communication, and promoting the highest quality of patient care. Defined as courteous and respectful behavior in interpersonal interactions, civility in medicine extends to relationships among healthcare providers, between doctors and patients, and within medical institutions. In an environment where stress and high-stakes decisions are commonplace, maintaining professionalism and respect is not just a matter of good etiquette it directly impacts patient outcomes, workplace morale, and the overall efficiency of the healthcare system (Fig. 3.1).

An 2022 article by Joel Geiderman and colleagues state; *that civil behavior is not only a good idea, but also a moral imperative for health care professionals* [1]. In defining Civility they refer to philosopher Cheshire Calhoun who wrote an article The Virtue of Civility in 2000; *in short, what makes being civil different from being respectful, considerate, or tolerant, is that civility always involves a display of respect, tolerance, or considerateness. Thus, civility is an essentially communicative form of moral conduct. In addition, because communicating our moral attitudes is central to civility, being genuinely civil—unlike, say, being genuinely considerate or genuinely tolerant—requires that we follow whatever the socially established norms are for showing people considerateness, tolerance, or respect. Only because there are such generally agreed upon, often codified, social rules for what counts as respectful, considerate, and tolerant behavior can we successfully communicate our moral attitudes toward others.. .. Similarly, incivilities draw on a common verbal and behavioral language for displaying disrespect, intolerance, or inconsiderateness* [2]. Geiderman's article notes that many studies have demonstrated that civility in inter-professional and therapeutic relationships is crucial to patient safety, quality of care, teamwork, and job satisfaction. Professor Forni describes four essential attributes in the meaning of civility these are: Civility is good, it is complex, it has to do with courtesy, politeness, and good manners, and belongs in the realm of ethics [3].

B. Silverman, *The Power of Bedside Manners in Patient Care*,
https://doi.org/10.1007/978-3-032-10496-0_3

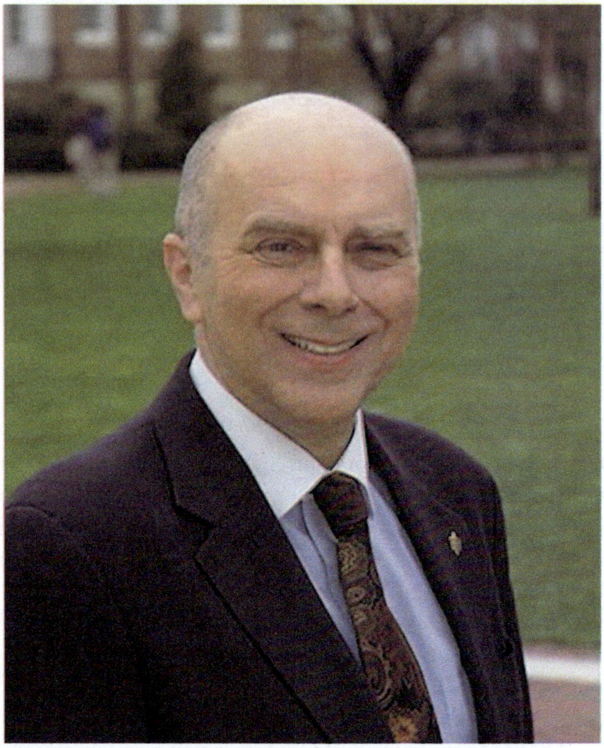

Fig. 3.1 P.M. Forni. (Courtesy of Johns Hopkins Magazine)The Johns Hopkins Professor whose book Choosing Civility: The Twenty-five Rules of Considerate Conduct is a guide to the value of civility in human relationship

Enhancing Patient Trust and Compliance

Patients enter medical settings often feeling vulnerable, anxious, and uncertain. Their trust in physicians and healthcare providers is built not only on technical expertise but also on the way they are treated. A civil and compassionate approach reassures patients, making them more likely to openly share critical health information, adhere to treatment plans, and engage in their own care. Studies have shown that when doctors communicate respectfully and empathetically, patient satisfaction and adherence to medical advice increase significantly. [4, 5] Conversely, dismissive or rude behavior can lead to misunderstandings, noncompliance, and even worse poor health outcomes.

Improving Teamwork and Collaboration

Modern medicine relies on teamwork, with physicians, nurses, technicians, and administrative staff working together to provide comprehensive care. Civility in these professional interactions fosters a collaborative environment where individuals feel valued and heard. When team members respect each other, they communicate more effectively, reducing errors and improving patient safety. Research has demonstrated that incivility, such as belittling colleagues or dismissing concerns, can lead to breakdowns in communication, medical errors, and compromised patient care [6]. By promoting civility, healthcare institutions create a culture of mutual respect that enhances both job satisfaction and patient outcomes. The issue of civil behavior has reached the point where the Joint Commission recommends that hospitals adopt policies for managing disruptive behavior. Examples include angry outbursts, rude acts, boundary violations, harassment, and profane or insulting language. It is likely your school, or institution has a code of conduct. Know it, respect it and follow it.

Reducing Burnout and Enhancing Workplace Well-Being

The medical profession is demanding, often requiring long hours, emotional resilience, and the ability to make life-or-death decisions under pressure. In such a high-stress environment, workplace incivility ranging from passive-aggressive remarks to overt hostility can contribute to burnout, emotional exhaustion, and job dissatisfaction. Studies indicate that medical professionals who experience disrespect or workplace bullying are more likely to suffer from mental health issues, disengagement, and even consider leaving the profession altogether. Conversely, a culture of civility supports emotional well-being, helping medical professionals feel supported and motivated in their work.

Preventing Medical Errors and Enhancing Patient Safety

Incivility in the medical field is not just a social concern it has direct implications for patient safety. Research has shown that rude or dismissive behavior can impair cognitive function, decrease problem-solving abilities, and increase the likelihood of medical errors. For instance, if a junior physician feels intimidated or dismissed by a senior colleague, they may hesitate to speak up about a potential mistake or a patient's deteriorating condition. Encouraging civility ensures that all team members feel comfortable voicing concerns, leading to better decision-making and ultimately safer patient care.

Forni's Most Important Rules

- Pay Attention
- Acknowledging others
- Speak and Act Kindly
- Respecting Boundaries, Time, and Space
- Think the Best and Assume good intentions
- Listen
- Be inclusive

- Respect and Give Praise
- Respect others' Opinions
- Apologize Earnestly
- Avoid Personal Questions
- Respect other People's Time
- Be Agreeable
- Don't Shift Responsibility and Blame

Conclusion

Civility in medicine is not a luxury but a necessity. It strengthens the patient-physician relationship, enhances teamwork, reduces burnout, and prevents medical errors. In an industry where lives are at stake, fostering an environment of respect and professionalism should be a top priority for healthcare institutions and individuals alike. By upholding civility, the medical community ensures that both patients and providers receive the care, respect, and dignity they deserve.

References

1. Geiderman JM, Moskop JC, Marco CA, Schears RM, Derse AR. Civility in health care: a moral imperative. EC Forum. 2022;36(2):245–57. https://doi.org/10.1007/s10730-022-09501-y.
2. Calhoun C. The virtue of civility. Philos Public Aff. 2000;29(3):251–75. https://doi.org/10.1111/j.1088-4963.2000.00251.x.
3. Forni RM. Mastering civility. New York: St. Martin's Griffin; 2002. p. 8–9.
4. Flickinger TF, Saha S, Roter D, Korthuis PT, Sharp V, Cohn J, et al. Respecting patients is associated with more patient-centered communication behaviors in clinical encounters. Patient Educ Couns. 2015;99(2):250–5. https://doi.org/10.1016/j.pec.2015.08.020.
5. Sharkiya SH. Quality communication can improve patient-centred health outcomes among older patients: a rapid review. BMC Health Serv Res. 2023;23:886. https://doi.org/10.1186/s12913-023-09869-8.
6. Voltz NB, Fringer R, Walters B, Kowalenko T. Prevalence of horizontal violence among emergency attending physicians, residents, and physician assistants. J Emerg Med. 2017;18(2):213–8. https://doi.org/10.5811/westjem.2016.10.31385.

Learning to Be Professional

4

The good physician treats the disease; the great physician treats the patient who has the disease. (Wm Osler)

From cranial nerves to the Krebs cycle, your medical education demands memorization of a vast landscape of facts and theories. You'll learn to diagnose, treat, and comfort patients, both in straightforward cases and complex ones. But beyond the science, medical professionalism is a way of being—a continuous process of becoming a better doctor. It's about 'practicing' medicine, not just doing it. Your journey into the medical profession begins with the transition from student to a bedside healthcare professional. This moment symbolizes your commitment to adopt the ethics, moral responsibilities, and professional standards that define medicine. Whether you chose medicine to help others, gain respect, or fulfill a personal dream, the donning of the White Coat sets you on a path toward professional growth and responsibility. The profession requires the acquisition and application of a body of knowledge and technical skills. You and your healthcare providers are bound together by shared commitment to heal the sick. In medicine this commitment is informed by scientific and clinical evidence but also considers the patients values and preferences [1] (Fig. 4.1).

B. Silverman, *The Power of Bedside Manners in Patient Care*,
https://doi.org/10.1007/978-3-032-10496-0_4

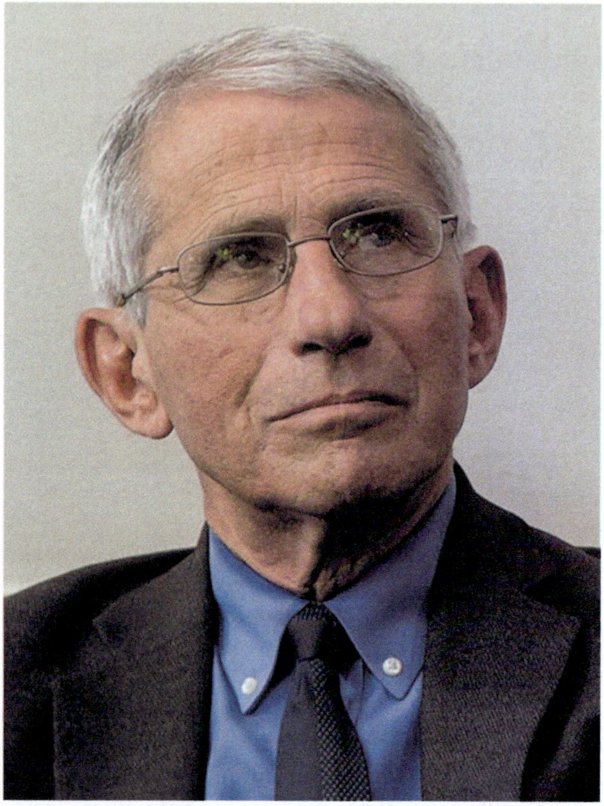

Fig. 4.1 Anthony FauciSpeaking on pandemics and public policy at Harvard Kennedy SchoolHe is an American physician scientist and immunologist who served as the director of the National Institute of Allergy and infectious Diseases. He is known for his courage, integrity, and professionalism. His conduct serves as a guide for all healthcare providers on the meaning of professionalism

Why Is Medical Professionalism Important

This statement in the article Understanding Medical Professionalism is an excellent description of why professionalism is necessary in medicine [2]. *Medicine is a complex system filled with uncertainties and ambiguities. The science is imperfect and complete with outcomes probabilistic at best. The knowledge and technology are vast and fast changing, such that almost impossible to master and sometimes make sense of it's appropriate use. Therapy must be instituted even when the diagnosis is incomplete. Even applying the scientific basis or evidence-based medicine does not result in certainty or predictability in clinical outcome. Professional judgment has always to be exercised in situations of incomplete information, resources and time. Illness makes patients vulnerable, anxious, depressed or fearful. Patients bring their own unique preferences expectations concerns biases and issues. Doctors working in teams are expected to communicate and perform consistently swiftly and humanely. Doctors, like all humans also have their own vulnerability and fallibility. Professionalism, as an ideology and applied physiology, provides a framework that allows stability and certainty in medical practice through the building of trust and confidence and patience and the sense of solidarity among all the stakeholders in medicine. The trust and confidence created by professionalism enables effective management of the uncertainty and complexity of medical practice, thus enabling healthcare professionals to meet the challenges and expectations of their work. The pillars of professionalism that promote and preserve trust and confidence in the healthcare system are marked by clinical competence, ethical competence, altruism and organizational professionalism in clinical and professional governance.*

Medical Professionalism Is Built on Four Core Ethical Principles

1. Autonomy: Respecting patients' rights to make informed decisions about their care.
2. **Non-malfeasance**: "Do no harm."
3. **Beneficence**: Acting in the best interest of the patient.
4. Social Justice: Ensuring fairness in medical care for all.

The Ten Professional Commitments [3]

1. Commitment to professional competence.
2. Commitment to honesty with patients.
3. Commitment to patient confidentiality.
4. Commitment to maintaining appropriate relations with patients.
5. Commitment to improving quality of care.
6. Commitment to improving access to care.
7. Commitment to just distribution of finite resources.
8. Commitment to scientific knowledge.
9. Commitment to maintaining trust by managing conflicts of interest.
10. Commitment to professional responsibilities.

These principles are the core of that it is to be a professional. A code that defines the relationship between doctors and society and emphasizes the importance of patient welfare as the most important component of professionalism.

Professionalism Beyond Skills

While medical knowledge and technical skills are essential, professionalism also demands certain attitudes and behaviors. The ideal healthcare professional is compassionate, honest, trustworthy, courageous, and committed to continuous learning. You saw this commitment during the COVID-19 pandemic where healthcare professionals around the world demonstrated these values working under extreme conditions and prioritizing patient care despite the risks. These principles are codified in the council for graduate medical education which lists requirements for professionalism as demonstrating respect, compassion, and integrity. Showing a responsiveness to the needs of patient and society. A commitment that supersedes self-interest and demonstrates accountability to patients, society, and our profession. They stress a commitment to ethical principles pertaining to the provision or withholding of clinical care, confidentiality of patient information, informed consent and business practices. And as a healthcare professional you must demonstrate sensitivity and responsiveness to the patient's culture, age, gender, and disabilities [4].

Patient Autonomy: A Vital Principle

Patient autonomy means empowering individuals to make informed decisions about their healthcare. Physicians must explain medical procedures, the potential risks and benefits, and, importantly, the costs. Using clear, understandable language is crucial to ensure patients are fully informed. Regular feedback from patients helps ensure they understand and are comfortable with their treatment plan.

The Philosophy of Medicine

Edmund Pellegrino, a key figure in medical ethics, argued that the ultimate goal of medicine is the good of the patient—acknowledging the patient's unique circumstances and needs. As a professional, your duty is not just to treat diseases but to restore or help individuals cope with illness in ways that respect their dignity.

The Hidden Curriculum: Learning Through Observation

Much of your development as a doctor happens not in textbooks, but in real-life interactions. You'll learn a lot from watching others—how your colleagues interact with patients and each other. Be an observant learner: recognize the behaviors that foster trust, empathy, and effective patient care, and avoid those that create unnecessary stress. Good bedside manners, like surgical skills, take practice and reflection. The danger of the hidden curriculum is the student will develop cynicism and learn bad habits on the wards. Students enter the wards with idealism but can be disillusioned when exposed to the hard work, dying patients, anxious families, and demanding supervisors. These experiences can undermine your efforts to be a true professional and it is important then you guard yourself against them and recognize those bedside competencies which promote professionalism and enhance patient care.

The Evolution of Medical Ethics

The ethical principles that guide modern medicine have deep roots in history. The Hippocratic Oath (circa 400 BCE) set the standard for physician behavior—emphasizing the importance of patient welfare, avoiding harm, and maintaining professional boundaries. This code influenced Christian philosophers, later updated by figures like John Gregory and Thomas Percival in the 18th and 19th centuries, who championed ethics such as benevolence and non-malfeasance. In response to the horrors of human experimentation in the twentieth century, ethical guidelines like the Nuremberg Code, Declaration of Helsinki, and the Belmont Code were established to protect human rights in research. These guidelines reinforce the importance of informed consent, the balance of risks and benefits, and respect for vulnerable populations.

The Changing Perception of Physicians

How society views physicians has shifted over the years. Once seen as epitomes of virtue, TV portrayals of doctors have evolved, reflecting broader cultural changes. In classic shows like Marcus Welby, M.D., doctors were portrayed as wise, compassionate figures. In contrast, modern depictions, such as House, often show doctors as flawed, self-centered, and even rude. These portrayals may not reflect reality, but they speak to a growing societal skepticism about authority figures, including healthcare providers. In medicine, professionalism is more than a set of rules—it's a lifelong commitment to improve, serve, and respect those who rely on your care. It's a balance of skill, compassion, and ethics, ensuring that the patient's well-being always comes first.

Chaperones and Patient Comfort

The physical exam is one of a physician's most critical tasks, but it's about more than just checking for disease—it's about making patients feel safe and understood. While patients may be physically naked during an exam, many also feel emotionally exposed. Whether they are struggling with illness, age, or body image, patients often feel vulnerable. A good physician must balance the need for a thorough exam with sensitivity to these emotions.

It's essential to create a comfortable, private, and well-lit environment. Exam rooms should be warm, and the atmosphere should be inviting, not rushed. While it's often necessary to have patients undress for a proper exam, this should be done with care—offering gowns instead of flimsy drapes and ensuring the patient's privacy and dignity are respected. Given the potential for inappropriate behavior in healthcare settings, it's vital to make sure patients feel safe during physical exams. it's advisable to have a chaperone present and this is especially encouraged with breast or genital examinations. Always document whether a patient wants a chaperone and respect their wishes. This ensures both patient comfort and legal protection for the physician.

The Physician Charter on Medical Professionalism

The following is drawn from the physician charter on medical professionalism. The charter that was created in 2002 by the American board of internal medicine foundation, the American College of physicians, the American Society of internal medicine, and the European federation of internal medicine [5, 6].

This document states that professionalism is the basis of medicine's contact with society. It demands placing the interests of patients above those of the physician, setting and maintaining standards of competence and integrity. Maintenance of the principles of professionalism are essential for the public to have trust in the medical profession, and this trust depends on the individual integrity of every physician.

The following are the fundamental principles of professionalism. The **first principle** is primacy of patient welfare. This requires that the health care provider is dedicated to serving the best interests of the patient. This altruism contributes to the trust that is central to health care provider physician-patient relationship. This relationship should not and cannot be compromised by market forces, administrative exigencies, or personal pressures. The **second principle** is patient autonomy. This requires that you are honest with your patients, and you empower them to make informed decisions concerning their treatment. This requires thoroughly addressing their concerns and answering their questions in a way that they can understand what you're planning. The **third principle** is social justice. It is important that you work actively to eliminate discrimination and bias whether it's based on gender, race, ethnicity, religion, or socioeconomic status. The **fourth principle** is to provide cost effective care. You have a commitment to just distribution of finite resources. You have a responsibility to order only those tests which will provide important diagnostic or therapeutic information for your patient and to offer your patient alternatives if the cost of testing or care exceeds their comfort level.

To maintain the patients' trust, it is essential that you manage conflicts of interest. This includes avoiding conflicts in your practice that result in private gain or personal advantage. You must be open and transparent when working with organizations that are for-profit industries, medical equipment manufacturers, insurance companies, and pharmaceutical firms. In your employment, you must be confident that your income is not based on financial incentives to do unnecessary testing or provide unneeded therapies [7].

As a physician or health care provider you must be committed to lifelong learning, and you are responsible for maintaining the medical knowledge and the clinical skills necessary for quality medical care. As a health care provider, you must ensure that the patients are completely and honestly informed before the consent to any treatment. You must answer all their questions and explain to them in terms that they can understand proposed treatments and therapies. You must explain to your patients the most significant and likely potential complications and side effects of proposed therapies.

Professionalism demands commitment to patient confidentiality. To earn their trust and confidence requires that you safeguard any personal or medical information that they provide. You are also committing to have appropriate relations with your patients. They are inherently vulnerable, dependent, and this requires then you maintain a strict professional relationship with them. This includes never exploiting your patients for sexual advantage, personal financial gain, or any private purpose. It is important that you were committed to the continuous improvement in the quality of your patient's health. This is not only about clinical competence but working collaboratively with other professionals to reduce medical error, increase patient safety, and minimize overuse of health care resources, and optimize the outcomes of their health care.

Your responsibility as a healthcare professional is not only to work with the individual patient but you must have a commitment to those professional societies that are committed to the improvement of our communities and your individual patient's health.

Prioritizing Patient Care over Personal Profit

But tell me, your physician in the precise sense of whom you were just speaking, is he a money maker, and earner of fees or healer of the sick? And remember to speak of the physician who really is such. (Plato (Republic341C))

Medicine is not merely a profession—it is a moral enterprise. At its core lies a profound ethical responsibility; to care for the vulnerable, to heal the affected, and to uphold the dignity of the human person. While financial compensation is a just and necessary part of a physician's livelihood, it must never eclipse the ultimate purpose of medical practice—the welfare of the patient.

The heart of this principle is the trust patients place in their physicians. A patient reveals their fears, their pains, and often their deepest vulnerabilities. This act of trust assumes that the doctor will act not out of self-interest, but in pursuit of the patients good. If a physician's decisions are swayed by profit— prescribing unnecessary treatments, favoring lucrative procedures, or limiting care to those who can pay—this sacred trust is broken.

This ethical imperative is echoed in the philosophy of Edmond Pellegrino, who viewed medicine as a covenant rather than a contract. For him the healing relationship is not a transaction but a moral bond. The patient, in a moment of weakness, appeals to the physician's knowledge and conscience—not their market calculations. Pellegrino insists *that the good of the patient is the ultimate end of medicine* and anything that subordinates this goal undermines both the practice and the practitioner.

In contrast, viewing medicine through purely economic lens risks commodifying the human person. The patient becomes a "consumer" and the doctor a "provider" reducing the richness of the healing relationship to a business exchange. This not only jeopardizes care quality but degrades the intrinsic dignity of both the patient and the physician.

Moreover, history offers powerful reminders of what is lost when profit prevails over principle. From medical scams to predatory insurance policies, each instance where money trump's care erodes public trust and inflames inequity. In contrast, physicians who championed the well-being of their patients—even at personal cost—embody the nobility of their calling. They remind us that healing is not just a science, but an art infused with empathy, courage, and moral clarity.

Ultimately, the measure of a great doctor is not in their salary, but in the lives they uplift, the dignity they preserve and the faith they honor. Medicine must never forget its true north; the patient, not the paycheck [8]. it is important to remember William Osler's advice; *the practice of medicine is an art, not a trade a calling, not a business; a calling in which your heart will be exercised equally with your head.*

Key Points

1. **Core Ethical Principles**:
   - **Patient Autonomy**: Respecting patients' right to make informed decisions.
   - **Nonmaleficence**: Avoiding harm to patients.
   - **Beneficence**: Acting in patients' best interest.
   - **Social Justice**: Fair distribution of healthcare resources.
2. **Historical Context**:
   - Rooted in the Hippocratic Oath, John Gregory's principles of humanity and sympathy, and Percival's 1803 Code of Medical Ethics.
   - The AMA Code (established in 1847) formalized ethical standards, aligning medicine with societal needs.
   - Developments like the Nuremberg Code (1947) and the Declaration of Helsinki (1964) established guidelines for ethical human research.
3. **Modern Challenges**:
   - Conflicts arise from balancing personal welfare, organizational demands, and ethical obligations.
4. **Practical Applications**:
   - Professional behavior must be modeled after bedside behaviors that promote patient trust.
   - Physicians must ensure transparency with patients about their conditions and treatments, even under challenging circumstances.
   - Respectful communication, empathy, and collaborative problem-solving are essential in clinical settings.
5. **The Role of Courage**:
   - The COVID-19 pandemic highlighted the importance of courage, as health-care workers prioritized patient care despite personal risks.

Medical professionalism is ultimately about upholding the patient's well-being above all else, integrating knowledge, ethics, and empathy into the practice of medicine.

References

1. Kirk LM. Professionalism in medicine: definitions and considerations for teaching. Proc (Bayl Univ Med Cent). 2007;20:13–6. https://doi.org/10.1080/08998280.2007.11928225.
2. Thirumoorthy T, Shelat VG. Understanding medical professionalism. Singapore Med J. 2025;66:114–8. https://doi.org/10.4103/singaporemedj.SMJ-2023-059. Epub 2025 Feb 17.
3. Blank L, Kimball H, McDonald W, Merino J. Medical professionalism in the new millennium. Ann Intern Med. 2003;138:839–41.
4. Accreditation Council for Graduate Medical Education. General competencies. Chicago: ACGME; 1999. Available from: www.acgme.org
5. ABIM Foundation, ACP–ASIM Foundation, European Federation of Internal Medicine. Medical professionalism in the new millennium: a physician charter. Ann Intern Med. 2002;136:243–6.
6. O'Gara PT, Ness DL, Harold JG. Medical professionalism and the American College of Cardiology: a renewed commitment. J Am Coll Cardiol. 2015;65:503–6.
7. Levison W, Ginsburg S, Hafferty FW, Lucey CR. Understanding medical professionalism. New York: McGraw-Hill; 2014.
8. Pellegrino ED. The commodification of medical and health care: the moral consequences of a paradigm shift from a professional to a market ethic. J Med Philos. 1999;24:243–66.

The Indispensable Role of Honesty in Medicine: Truth-Telling Is a Cornerstone of the Physician Patient Relationship

5

Honesty—defined as transparency, truthfulness, and integrity in communication and action—is the bedrock of medical practice. It underpins patient trust, ensures informed consent, strengthens teamwork, mitigates harm, and upholds the profession's moral foundation. In an era of complex treatments and heightened patient autonomy, honesty is not just virtuous but vital to ethical, effective care [1] (Fig. 5.1).

Patient Trust and Autonomy

Honesty begins with the patient-physician relationship. Patients entrust clinicians with their vulnerabilities, relying on truthful information to make life-altering decisions. Clinical studies have found that patients who perceived their doctors as honest were significantly more likely to adhere to treatment plans. A physician who candidly explains a cancer prognosis—including uncertainties—empowers the patient to weigh palliative care versus aggressive therapy. Conversely, evasiveness or sugarcoating risks eroding trust, leading to disengagement or resentment. Honesty respects patient autonomy, a pillar of medical ethics, ensuring individuals retain control over their bodies and futures.

Informed Consent and Shared Decision-Making

Informed consent, legally and ethically mandated, hinges on honesty. A surgeon outlining a procedure's risks—even rare complications like paralysis—enables patients to consent meaningfully. Honesty here is not merely reciting a script but engaging in dialogue. For instance, a psychiatrist prescribing antidepressants must transparently discuss side effects, withdrawal risks, and alternatives. This openness fosters collaboration, aligning care with patient values and reducing litigation [2].

B. Silverman, *The Power of Bedside Manners in Patient Care*,
https://doi.org/10.1007/978-3-032-10496-0_5

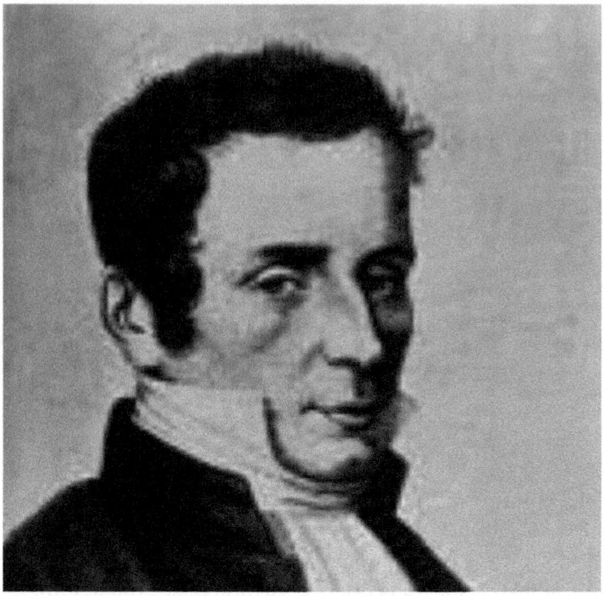

Fig. 5.1 Rene Laennec from the Wellcome CollectionHe invented the stethoscope in 1816 and revolutionized medicine by introducing the first technology to diagnosis disease. As a physician he was known for his integrity and commitment to science

Courts increasingly penalize nondisclosure, emphasizing honesty as both a moral and legal duty.

Team Collaboration and Professional Integrity

Honesty sustains teamwork in medicine. Miscommunication among nurses, specialists, and pharmacists accounts for nearly 70% of hospital errors, per a 2019 Joint Commission report. A culture of honesty—where a nurse feels safe to question a dosage or a resident admits uncertainty—prevents harm. Professionally, honesty also combats toxic hierarchies. Mentors who openly share past mistakes, like misdiagnoses, model accountability, nurturing a culture of growth over blame.

Error Disclosure and Ethical Accountability in Medicine

Mistakes are an unfortunate but inevitable part of medical practice. However, the way clinicians respond to these errors can profoundly influence their impact. When a healthcare provider openly admits to an error—whether it's a missed diagnosis or a surgical complication—and offers a sincere apology, patients are far more likely to respond with understanding and forgiveness.

Ethically, transparency reflects the core principle of the Hippocratic Oath: "do no harm." Hiding mistakes often does greater damage—patients may miss out on timely corrective care, and clinicians may experience moral distress. The harm of concealment is both clinical and emotional.

To guide ethical and effective disclosure, several best practices have been developed. At the heart of these is the need to build trust, which includes:

Clinical Support

Ensure patients have prompt access to their medical records. Arrange any necessary follow-up tests, treatments, or referrals to address the consequences of the error.

Respect and Communication

Prepare carefully for disclosure conversations. Actively listen and engage with empathy, taking time to understand the patient's perspective. Whenever possible, involve staff who know the patient and can offer continuity and compassionate support.

Emotional and Practical Support

Disclosing an error isn't just a single conversation—it's a process. Offer continued emotional support through counselors, social workers, or support groups. You may also need to help with logistical issues such as medical record access or covering reasonable costs associated with the error.

Encourage questions and be ready to provide clear, honest answers. This openness helps patients feel respected and less alone in navigating the fallout.

Analysis and Improvement

Every disclosure should be followed by a serious internal review of the event. What went wrong? How can care be improved? Patients deserve to know how systems are being strengthened to prevent similar incidents.

Two excellent resources for guidance include:

- **The Canadian Disclosure Guidelines: Being Open with Patients and Families**, which offers detailed steps for transparent and compassionate communication [3].
- **The Massachusetts Coalition for the Prevention of Medical Errors' guide**, *When Things Go Wrong: Responding to Adverse Events*, which emphasizes two principles: medical care must be **safe** and **patient centered** [4].

These guidelines stress that patients and families have the right to know what happened and how it may affect them. Communication should be open, timely—ideally within 24 h—and ongoing. Avoid defensive or legalistic tones, which often deepen mistrust and emotional pain.

A helpful question for any clinician is: *If I were harmed by my care, how would I want to be told?*

The Massachusetts Coalition Recommends Four Key Steps

1. **Tell the patient and family what happened.** Save detailed explanations of causes or systemic issues for a follow-up conversation.
2. **Take responsibility.** The attending physician should acknowledge the error without deflecting blame.
3. **Offer a sincere apology.** Authenticity matters more than perfectly crafted words.
4. **Outline next steps.** Explain how care will continue and what measures will be taken to prevent similar incidents in the future.

Good communication, empathy, and accountability not only reduce stress and anxiety but also preserve the therapeutic relationship. Mistakes happen. It's how we respond that defines the ethics—and humanity—of care.

Public Health and Research Integrity

Beyond individual care, honesty safeguards public health. During crises like COVID-19, transparent communication about vaccine efficacy or supply shortages builds public cooperation. Conversely, dishonesty fuels distrust; the Tuskegee Syphilis Study's deceit, for instance, left enduring scars in Black communities. Similarly, research fraud—such as falsified data in drug trials—jeopardizes lives and undermines scientific progress. Honest reporting of trial outcomes, even when unfavorable, ensures treatments are safe and evidence based.

Conclusion

Honesty in medicine is not passive truth-telling but an active commitment to integrity. It bridges the gap between clinician expertise and patient agency, transforms errors into lessons, and fortifies healthcare's moral compass. In a world of AI diagnostics and personalized medicine, honesty remains irreplaceable—a reminder that medicine's power lies not in perfection but in its humanity. Cultivating honesty requires institutional support: training in communication, protections for whistleblowers, and policies prioritizing transparency over liability fears. As physician-writer Abraham Verghese noted, "The patient's story is the beating heart of medicine." Honesty ensures that story is heard, respected, and honored.

References

1. Hart JL. Deception, honesty, and professionalism: a persistent challenge in modern medicine. Curr Opin Psychol. 2022;47:101434. https://doi.org/10.1016/j.copsyc.2022.101434.
2. Huntington B, Kuhn N. Communication gaffes: a root cause of malpractice claims. Proc (Bayl Univ Med Cent). 2003;16:2003157–61.
3. Canadian disclosure guidelines: being open with patients and families. Edmonton: Canadian Patient Safety Institute; 2011. ISBN 9781926541389.
4. Powell SK. The Massachusetts Coalition for the Prevention of Medical Errors' guide, when things go wrong: responding to adverse events. Jt Comm J Qual Improv. 2006;32:379–83. https://doi.org/10.1097/00129234-200607000-00001.

Listening to the Patient

6

Listening: The Foundation of Good Manners in Medicine

At the heart of good manners in medicine is the art of listening. Patients must feel heard, especially when discussing complex or sensitive health concerns. A doctor who listens attentively creates a safe space where patients feel comfortable sharing their worries without fear of judgment or interruption. This practice goes beyond merely collecting information; it's about fostering rapport and building trust. Dr. Philip Tumulty, in a 1978 speech to the Johns Hopkins medical students called "The Art of Healing," gave them this advice; "*A clinician must be patient and forbearing, strong yet gentle, unselfish of his time and unstinting in his efforts. He must be willing to bite his tongue and to turn his cheek. He must have an attentive ear as well as the ability to question probingly. His attitude must create trust and confidence, and his manner thoughtfulness and security. He must hear what the patient doesn't say and be sensitive to the anguish which cannot be expressed. Patients are anxious; they are frightened; they inwardly anticipate the very worst, although they may cover up with apparent lack of concern. Some are very brave, while others cling in terror. All grasp tightly to life, and in all, some glimmer of hope, no matter how flickering, is essential to the vitality of their spirit*" (Fig. 6.1).

It's not just about medical expertise; it's about showing patients that you care. Good bedside manners reflect a commitment to quality care and are integral to the healing process. By prioritizing civility, empathy, and attentiveness, you can foster trust, enhance communication, and ultimately provide better care. Though not every patient can be cured, the simple act of showing respect can significantly impact their experience and recovery.

B. Silverman, *The Power of Bedside Manners in Patient Care*,
https://doi.org/10.1007/978-3-032-10496-0_6

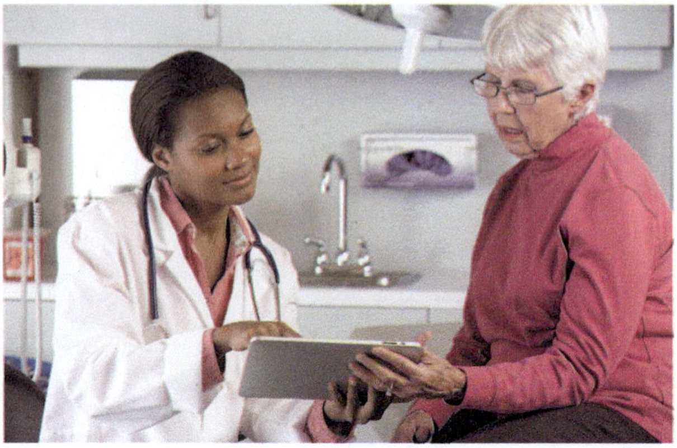

Fig. 6.1 Medical student engaged and listening to a patient

Building Trust in Patient Care

Trust is the cornerstone of the doctor-patient relationship. But how do patients determine if they can trust you? They can't assess your medical skills or medical knowledge directly. Instead, they often rely on recommendations, online reviews, and the doctor's credentials. However, the most significant factor in establishing trust is your behavior—specifically, your bedside manner. They can judge how well you listen, communicate, and treat them with respect.

The overall environment plays a role too. A well-kept office, polite staff, contribute to a positive impression. Office wait times, the demeanor of the staff, and the comfort of the waiting and exam rooms all matter in making patients feel welcome and cared for. Patients expect a high standard of professionalism from both the doctor and their team. A guide is this comment from George Beller, former chief of cardiology at the University of Virginia: "*The patient should expect the physician to be caring and empathetic, take the time to explain what was found in the medical evaluation, describe the disease process in lay terms, not hurry when answering questions, show sensitivity and compassion when having to relate bad news, display a realistic but positive attitude about treatment plans, and fully explain why certain tests are being ordered and specific drugs or procedures are being recommended*".

Dr. David Pendleton and co-authors, in the book *The New Consultation: Developing Doctor-Patient Communication* [1], state the doctor must: (a) understand the problem, (b) understand the patient, (c) the doctor and the patient must agree on the problem, (d) share decisions and responsibility, and (e) maintain a relationship. Effective consultations leave patients with a clear understanding of their diagnosis, treatment plan, and next steps. When doctors engage with patients, listen to their concerns, and offer clear explanations, patients are more likely to follow medical advice. Non-verbal communication also plays a critical role in building trust. Facial expressions, body language, and attentiveness all contribute to how patients perceive their care. Dr. Jerome Groopman, in *How Doctors Think*, stresses that allowing patients to tell their full story fosters mutual respect and trust—both of which are essential for successful treatment outcomes.

The Healthcare-Patient Relationship

The healthcare provider-patient relationship has evolved, especially with the rise of technology and compartmentalized care. While diagnostic tools like CT scans and MRIs are invaluable, they cannot replace the trust and connection fostered through direct, personal interaction. Trust is built through face-to-face contact, attentive listening, and empathy. Dr. Bernard Lown wrote in *The Lost Art of Healing* that empathy, attentiveness, and caring are essential for restoring the doctor-patient relationship. Effective communication is key to earning trust—but this doesn't just mean answering questions. It means listening deeply and giving patients the space to express their concerns without interruption. Studies show that doctors often interrupt the patient's story within the first 23 s of the consultation. When patients don't feel heard, they lose confidence in the doctor's conclusions. Dr. William T. Branch, Jr., a professor of medicine at Emory University School of Medicine, demonstrated that faculty members coached on issues such as how to listen carefully, how to be a caring person, and how to use personal and social information in patient care were better at teaching these skills to medical students than faculty who had not been coached. Dr. Branch pointed out that the skills taught to the faculty "can help physicians grow, not just in terms of knowing more but in becoming a whole person" [2, 3].

Reflecting on his own hospital care, Dr. Michael Kahn, a psychiatrist writing in the *The New England Journal of Medicine*, noted that while compassion is preferred, most patients would be well served with a doctor who is well behaved. He wrote about his attending surgeon:

> *I found the Old World manners of my European born surgeon—and my reaction to them—revealing in this regard. Whatever he might actually have been feeling, his behavior—dress, manners, body language, eye contact—was impeccable. I wasn't left thinking 'What compassion.' Instead I found myself thinking, 'What a professional,' and even (unexpectedly) 'What a gentleman.' The impression he made was remarkably calming, and it helped to confirm my suspicion that patients may care less about whether their doctors are reflective and empathetic than whether they are respectful and attentive.* [4]

Conclusion

For a doctor-patient relationship to be effective, trust must be built on clear communication, empathy, and respect. Healthcare providers who listen attentively, provide clear explanations, and maintain professionalism foster lasting trust with their patients. As the healthcare system continues to evolve, it's essential that you do not lose sight of the human connection at the heart of healing. Trust remains the foundation of good patient care, and it can be nurtured through every interaction.

References

1. Pendleton D, Schofield T, Tate P, Havelock P. The new consultation: developing doctor–patient communication. Oxford: Oxford University Press; 2003. https://doi.org/10.1093/med/9780192632883.001.0001.
2. Branch WT Jr. Teaching compassion. Patient Educ Couns. 2012;89:3–4. https://doi.org/10.1016/j.pec.2012.03.013. Epub 2012 May 10.
3. Branch WT Jr, Kern D, Haidet P, Weissmann P, Gracey CF, Mitchell G, Inui T. The patient–physician relationship: teaching the human dimensions of care in clinical settings. JAMA. 2001;286(9):1067–74. https://doi.org/10.1001/jama.286.9.1067.
4. Kahn M. Etiquette-based medicine. N Engl J Med. 2008;358:1988–9.

7 Empathy and Aequanimitas: Vital Concepts in Medicine to Understand and Bring to the Bedside

Treat the Soul

In halls where anxious hearts reside,
A doctor walks with steady stride.
Not just with knowledge, sharp and clear,
But words that calm, and ears that hear.

He speaks with kindness, soft and true,
In every glance, respect shines through.
Patient tales, he holds with care,
Their dignity his sacred prayer.

No rushed glance, no hurried note,
But presence warm, like gentle coat.
Building trust with every breath,
A healer's art that knows no death.

For more than body, bone, or pain,
He treats the soul, where fears remain.
A beacon bright, both wise and just—
A doctor earned their patient's trust.

Empathy in Medicine: A Vital, Human Connection

Empathy isn't just a nice-to-have in medicine—it's a clinical superpower. It's the ability to understand and share another person's feelings, allowing healthcare providers to truly connect with patients on a human level [1]. Far from being just an emotional response, empathy plays a crucial role in improving patient outcomes, building trust, and creating a more compassionate healthcare environment [2] (Fig. 7.1).

B. Silverman, *The Power of Bedside Manners in Patient Care*,
https://doi.org/10.1007/978-3-032-10496-0_7

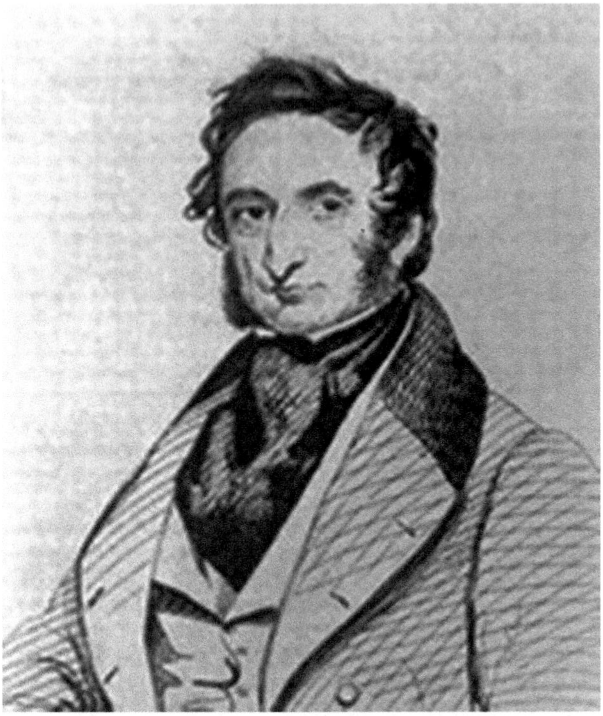

Fig. 7.1 Robert Graves from the Welcome Institute CollectionHe was an Irish physician who reformed medical education. His approach emphasized bedside teaching over abstract lectures. He had a lasting influence especially his approach to bedside teaching, interacting with the patient, and caring for the individual as a person

As neuroscientist Jean Decety noted in a 2020 *American Journal of Medicine* review, "empathy" is a relatively new term used to describe a wide range of psychological and physiological phenomena—from simply recognizing another's emotions to being motivated to help them [3]. In clinical practice, it often means tuning into a patient's experience through subtle verbal and non-verbal cues, adopting their perspective, and letting them know they've been seen and heard. This is what Decety calls **cognitive empathy**—the deliberate effort to step into someone else's shoes and understand their subjective experience.

Why Empathy Matters to Patients

When physicians listen with empathy, something powerful happens—patients open-up. They're more likely to share important symptoms, fears, and concerns, which can lead to more accurate diagnoses and better treatment outcomes. One study in *Academic Medicine* even found that patients treated by empathetic doctors had faster recoveries and were more likely to stick to their treatment plans [4]. Why? Because empathy builds trust — and trust makes people more willing to follow medical advice and actively participate in their own care.

Empathy also helps reduce the emotional toll of illness. Facing a frightening diagnosis or undergoing a painful procedure is overwhelming for many patients.

A provider who offers not just clinical expertise but also compassion and understanding can ease those feelings of fear and vulnerability. Imagine a cancer patient being told their diagnosis: the facts matter, yes—but so does the way they're delivered. A caring voice and a kind word can make a world of difference.

The Doctor-Patient Relationship: Built on Empathy

Empathy strengthens the doctor-patient relationship—the foundation of high-quality care. This is especially vital in managing chronic conditions like diabetes, heart disease, or depression, where ongoing communication and trust are essential. Patients who feel genuinely cared for are more likely to stay engaged in their treatment and motivated to make difficult lifestyle changes. Simply put, empathy helps keep the healing partnership strong.

What About the Doctors?

Interestingly, empathy doesn't just help patients—it helps clinicians, too. Doctors and nurses who practice empathy often report greater job satisfaction and a deeper sense of purpose. In a profession known for long hours, emotional stress, and burnout, empathy can serve as a kind of psychological buffer. It reminds providers *why* they chose medicine in the first place.

Can Empathy Be Dangerous? Understanding Aequanimitas

That said, there's a line. Too much emotional involvement—known as **emotional empathy**—can lead to **compassion fatigue**, a state of emotional exhaustion where providers become overwhelmed by the suffering of others [5]. This can blur the boundaries between self and patient, eventually leading to detachment, decreased performance, and burnout [6]. Balance is key: healthcare professionals must learn to connect deeply without losing themselves in the process.

Your relationship with the patient can become toxic when you develop such a close connection to the patient that the patient's motives and feeling are more of an effort to please their physician than to identify their own feelings and sentiment to adjust their illness in a manner that most reflects their own wishes. I experienced this when a patient with severely decompensated end stage heart failure came to the hospital. His physician was not on call, and they were very close. The patient shared with me that he was exhausted and ready to die but fought on to please his doctor. Now with his doctor not present, he finally felt he could yield to the disease.

William Osler addressed this issue in his address to the graduating medical class at the University of Pennsylvania in May of 1889. Titled "Aequanimitas" he recommended the following doctor patient relationship [7].

Osler urged physicians to develop **aequanimitas**, which he described as "coolness and presence of mind under all circumstances." He believed that doctors must learn to stay composed in the face of suffering, chaos, or uncertainty, so they could make clear decisions and offer steady leadership [8].

Imperturbability

In the physician or surgeon no quality takes rank with imperturbability. Osler used the term "imperturbability" to describe a kind of unflappable calm—not indifference, but rather disciplined restraint in emotion. A physician must feel compassion, he argued, but not become overwhelmed by emotion. "The serene judgment in moments of grave peril, the calm attitude in emergencies, the quiet grasp of the situation... are the qualities which count."

Detached Concern

He also spoke of "a certain measure of insensibility"—a controversial but important idea. He did not mean heartlessness, but rather the mental discipline to maintain objectivity. A good doctor must learn how to care deeply but not break down emotionally every time a patient suffers or dies.

The Physician's Burden

Osler acknowledged that this emotional balance was not easy and came only with experience and reflection. Young doctors might struggle with being too emotionally involved, but over time, they would learn the value of calm detachment as a tool of professional compassion.

Teaching Empathy: A Skill, Not Just a Trait

The good news? Empathy can be taught. Medical schools and residency programs are beginning to treat empathy not just as a personality trait but as a skill—one that can be developed through training. Role-playing scenarios, reflective writing, and guided patient interactions are just a few of the ways schools are helping future doctors become not just competent clinicians, but compassionate caregivers [9].

In Conclusion

Empathy is more than just a warm feeling—it's a critical tool for effective medical care. It improves patient outcomes, reduces anxiety, strengthens trust, and enhances professional fulfillment. But it also demands emotional awareness and self-care to avoid burnout. By recognizing the power—and limits—of empathy, the medical field can create a more humane, healing, and sustainable healthcare system for everyone involved. Osler's Aequanimitas is a call for the physician to develop strength of character, balancing compassion with emotional steadiness. His message continues to influence medical professionalism today, reminding doctors that how they carry themselves—not just what they know—shapes the quality of care they give.

References

1. Spiro HM. What is empathy and can it be taught? In: Spiro H, McCrea Curnen MG, Peschel E, St. James D, editors. Empathy and the practice of medicine. New Haven: Yale University Press; 1993. p. 7–14.
2. Mercer SW, Reynolds WJ. Empathy and quality of care. Br J Gen Pract. 2002;52:S9–12.
3. Decety J. Empathy in medicine: what it is, and how much we really need it. Am J Med. 2020;133:561–6.
4. Hojat M, Louis DZ, Markham FW, et al. Physicians' empathy and clinical outcomes for diabetic patients. Acad Med. 2011;86(3):359–64.
5. Zenasni F, Boujut E, Woerner A, Sultan S. Burnout and empathy in primary care: three hypotheses. Br J Gen Pract. 2012;62:346–7. https://doi.org/10.3399/bjgp12X652193.
6. Samra R. Empathy and burnout in medicine—acknowledging risks and opportunities. J Gen Intern Med. 2018;33:991–3. https://doi.org/10.1007/s11606-018-4443-5.
7. Bryan CS. Aequanimitas revisited. J S C Med Assoc. 1995;91:355–8.
8. Young JB. Does Osler's "aequanimitas" inform our contemporary pursuit of stillness? AMA J Ethics. 2022;24:E1166–71.
9. Batt-Rawden SA, Chisholm MS, Anton B, Flickinger TF. Teaching empathy to medical students: an updated, systematic review. Acad Med. 2013;88:1171–7. https://doi.org/10.1097/ACM.0b013e318299f3e3.

Preserving Human Dignity in Clinical Care

8

In this book there had been considerable discussion concerning supporting the dignity and humanity of an individual. But what does that really mean in this age of biotechnology, artificial intelligence, and genomics. In a book Human Dignity and Bioethics edited by Edmund D Pellegrino, Adam Shulman, and Thomas W Merrill [1]. Doctor Pellegrino has a chapter discussing the significance of dignity in medicine. It is helpful for you to consider his words when you were caring for a patient and involved in life saving and life changing decisions (Fig. 8.1).

B. Silverman, *The Power of Bedside Manners in Patient Care*,
https://doi.org/10.1007/978-3-032-10496-0_8

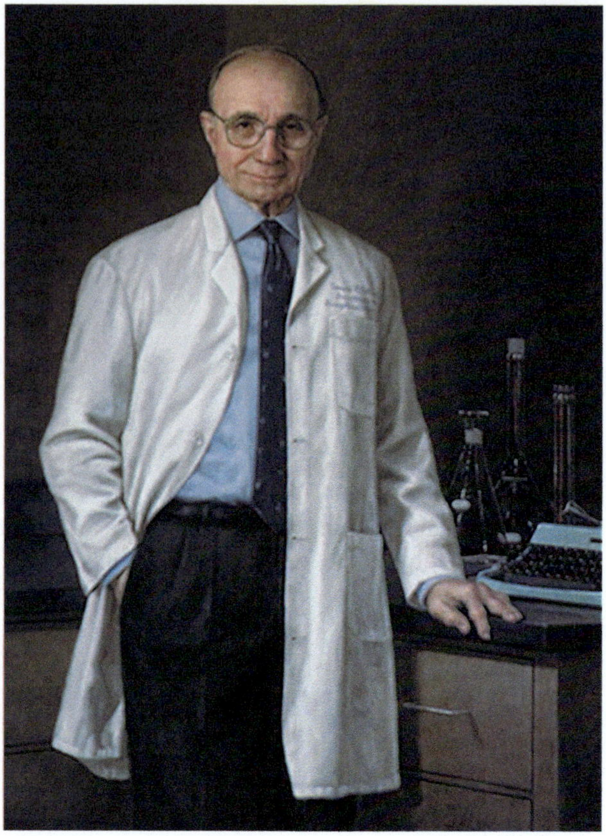

Fig. 8.1 Edmund Pellegrino. (Portrait by Jerry Crowley Bioethicist and medical Philosopher)

Intrinsic Dignity: The Foundation of Moral Worth

Intrinsic dignity refers to the inherent worth that every human being possesses simply by virtue of being human. It is:

- Universal and unchanging
- Independent of status, abilities, or opinion
- The grounding for human rights and moral entitlements

This principle is enshrined in the **1948 Universal Declaration of Human Rights** and the **UNESCO Declaration on Bioethics and Human Rights**, both of which place human dignity as the bedrock of all rights and ethical responsibilities.

Extrinsic Dignity: Society's Measure of Worth

In contrast, extrinsic dignity is socially constructed. It is:

- Based on perceived attributes like behavior, status, appearance, or group identity
- Vulnerable to praise or judgment from others—or from oneself
- Gained or lost through social approval, legal systems, or cultural norms

Pellegrino notes that we are constantly—consciously and unconsciously—making judgments about our own dignity and that of others. These judgments are shaped by interactions within our communities. Ultimately, we experience dignity not in isolation, but through encounters with others.

The Clinical Encounter: A Crucible of Dignity

Dr. Pellegrino defines the clinical encounter as a face-to-face meeting between a healer and a person in need of healing. This moment is more than a medical transaction—it is an ethical and existential exchange. The patient, in asking for help, exposes their vulnerability. They risk being seen as weak, dependent, or diminished. This loss of autonomy can feel like a threat to their extrinsic dignity. Pellegrino observes that: *Merely admitting the need for help places a person in a state of vulnerability... how that vulnerability is received determines whether the patient's dignity is sustained or undermined.* A good physician understands that the clinical relationship is inherently unequal—in knowledge, power, and control. It is precisely this imbalance that demands *greater moral responsibility* from the clinician.

Restoring Dignity in Times of Suffering

When patients are suffering, disfigured, or dying, they may lose confidence in their own dignity. Some may even feel guilt for being ill—blaming themselves and perceiving their condition as a personal failure. This is where the physician's role becomes especially crucial: not just to treat disease, but to affirm the patient's enduring worth. To reassure the patient, authentically and consistently, that they are still worthy of time, attention, and care—right to the very end.

The Moral Trust in Medicine

Pellegrino argues that the preservation of human dignity is not optional—it is central to the moral purpose of medicine. When physicians act with arrogance or indifference, they betray this moral trust. He warns against the intoxicating pride that can accompany the physician's power—particularly among the young and dangerously entrenched in older practitioners. When self-importance replaces humility, the physician risks prioritizing their own ego over the patient's good. To truly honor a patient's dignity, physicians must be:

- Present and available—including meeting with patients or families when asked
- Realistic yet compassionate—avoiding false hope or avoidance of difficult truths
- Advocates for dignity—supporting patients emotionally and morally, not just physically

Even at the end of life, the physician's role is critical. They help patients and families confront mortality, make decisions about hospice care, and accept the limits of medicine—while still affirming the patient's intrinsic value.

A Call to Compassionate Presence

Pellegrino reminds us that dignity is preserved not only through grand gestures, but through small acts of presence, kindness, and honesty. When a physician listens, takes time, answers questions, and acknowledges suffering, they restore a patient's sense of self. He also urges physicians to help families understand how to respond to the patient's vulnerability with respect—reinforcing the patient's pride, rather than unintentionally deepening their sense of loss.

Conclusion

In an age of dazzling technology and clinical efficiency, Pellegrino calls us back to the bedrock of care: seeing the patient as a person, affirming their worth, and defending their dignity—especially when it's at risk. His message is clear: *The true measure of a physician is not found in technical mastery alone, but in the ability to be fully human in the presence of another's suffering.*

Reference

1. Pellegrino ED. Chapter 20 The lived experience of human dignity. In: Pellegrino ED, Schulman A, Merrill TW, editors. Human dignity and bioethics. Notre Dame: University of Notre Dame Press; 2009.

Spiritualityin Medicine: Addressing Spiritual Needs in Clinical Practice

9

Spirituality can be defined as the way one feels towards the transcendental questions of meaning of life and our search for purpose and value. The religious sense is to be born of God, surrendered and obedient to the holy spirit [2] Many of your patients have strong spiritual beliefs and to ignore them is disrespectful.

To understand a patient's spirituality, health care providers must first take a careful spiritual history. This includes using tools like FICA which stands for faith, importance, community, and addressing spiritually in the patient's care [3]. When considering f**aith**, you can ask a patient do you consider yourself spiritual or religious. Then ask what **importance** your spirituality has in your life or in making health care decisions. Are you part of a religious or spiritual **community**? How would you like me, as your health care provider to **address** these issues in your care (Fig. 9.1).

You must listen to the patient with empathy and respect, avoid assumptions, be open to each patients' unique world view, and show genuine interest and support without imposing your own beliefs. You need to be able to recognize signs of spiritual distress. Patients may show this through a sense of hopelessness, anger at God or their fate, feelings of meaninglessness, fear of being a burden, feeling guilt or facing unresolved issues in their lives.

Responsibility as a Healthcare Provider

Your role as a health care professional is not to be their religious chaplain. But still, you must acknowledge and respect their spirituality as a legitimate and important part of that patient's identity. This would include supporting referrals to chaplains, clergy or spiritual counselors if the patient or their family request this counseling. You might be willing to integrate spiritual concerns into your care plan especially when this is palliative and end of life care. This support will affirm the patient's dignity, sense of control, and sources of strength. It is important to respect the

B. Silverman, *The Power of Bedside Manners in Patient Care*,
https://doi.org/10.1007/978-3-032-10496-0_9

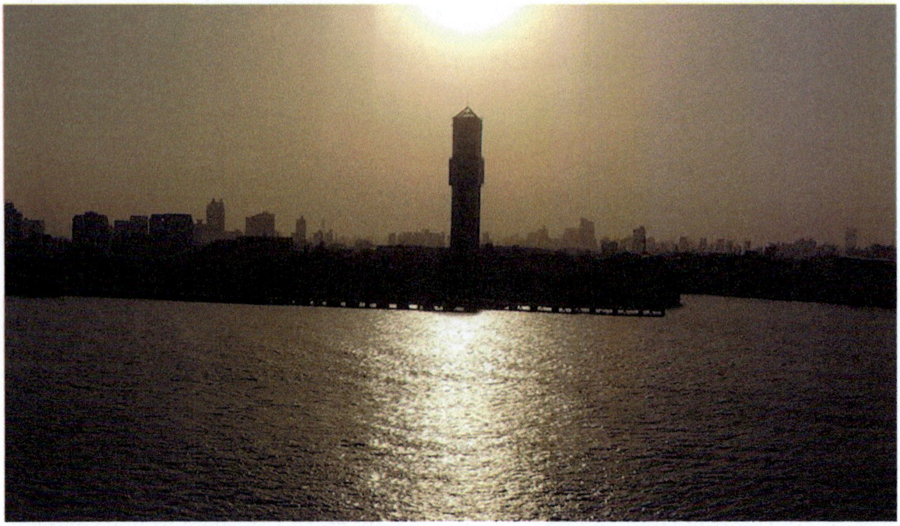

Fig. 9.1 *Mind, body, and soul are inseparable. Throughout human history, healing has been regarded as a spiritual event. Illness especially serious illness inevitably raises questions beyond science questions of a transcendental nature.* [1] (Daniel Sulmasy, Georgetown professor in the Kennedy Institute of Ethics)

patient's cultural background and religious beliefs, even if they differ from your own. You're not there to impose your own personal beliefs always ask rather than assume and create a safe nonjudgmental space for spiritual expression. You must remember that healing goes beyond curing. Even in incurable conditions spiritual care can help patients find peace, reconciliation or forgiveness and help strengthen relationships with loved ones. You must be willing to support a sense of legacy or meaning and foster acceptance and dignity at the end of life.

Understanding a patient's spirituality means recognizing that medical care must engage the whole person mind, body, and spirit. When honoring spiritual dimensions, the healthcare provider becomes more humane, responsive, and truly healing. It affirms even in illness and suffering that there is value in the patient's story, beliefs, and sense of purpose.

Clinical Case Example

Consider the following clinical example, Mrs. S, a 75-year-old woman with advanced metastatic breast cancer. She was recently admitted with complications of shortness of breath, fatigue, and weight loss. Her prognosis is poor, and the oncology team recommends transitioning to hospice care. But Mrs. S is hesitant to stop aggressive treatment. She says, "I believe if I have enough faith God will heal me." The care team feels that this is unrealistic expectation, but they want to respect her beliefs and affirm her dignity. They consult the hospital chaplain, and the attending physician uses the FICA rule at the bedside as he discusses with her the plan of care.

F in the rule stands for faith and Mrs. **S** is a devout Christian and very active in her church. **A** stands for importance and her faith gives her strength and hope and she does believe that miracles can happen. The **C** stands for her church community which she visits often and is of tremendous support for her emotionally. And the **A** means that she wants her care team to address her faith and belief and respect that she believed healing is possible.

It is important that the care team acknowledge that her faith is important to her, and they are willing to support her in any way they can. This means not just physically but emotionally and spiritually.

Her physician says, "let's talk about healing, even if it doesn't mean curing the disease." He asked her to work with a palliative care team to explore a peaceful and meaningful transition to her life. With this support, Mrs. S agrees to hospice care and did not frame it as giving up but trusting that God will prioritize her comfort and peace and maybe bring a cure for her. She finds emotional relief through prayer and pastoral support and she's able to express that she's at peace knowing that her faith and dignity were honored in the final stages of her life.

Recognizing her spirituality provided meaning and resilience but it also was important in shaping medical choices. It allowed for an open respectful conversation that helped integrate faith and medicine without conflict. It improved her trust in the health care team and allowed for communication and satisfaction for the patient and the family.

We understand from this example that spiritual care in medicine isn't about promoting any relief system, it's about listening deeply to what matters most to the patient and recognizing that healing isn't always physical but must allow space for hope, meaning and peace even in a dying patient.

References

1. Sulmasy DP. Physicians, spirituality, and compassionate patient care. N Engl J Med. 2024;390:1061–3. https://doi.org/10.1056/NEJMp231049.
2. The Holy Bible, John 1:12–13; John 3:5–8; 1 John 4:7.
3. FICA Spiritual Assessment Tool. Coalition for compassionate care of California. Available from: https://coalitionccc.org/CCCC/CCCC/Resources/FICA-Spiritual-Assessment-Tool.aspx. Accessed 15 Aug 2025.

Beyond the White Coat: The Art of Making a Lasting First Impression

10

The way you present yourself—through appearance and body language—has a powerful impact on how others perceive you. In fact, people form first impressions within seconds, often before you even speak [1]. In healthcare, where trust and connection are essential, these impressions can strongly influence a patient's comfort, confidence, and willingness to engage.

Hippocratic Thought on Physician Appearance

We begin with the Greeks in the fourth century BC, as does almost everything in Western culture. Physicians like Hippocrates were often indistinguishable from philosophers—robes or togas, no special attire. The emphasis was on wisdom, not appearance. The Greeks were very specific about physician bedside manners. Included in the Hippocratic corpus is this comment: *The physician ought also to be confidential, very chaste, sober, not a winebibber, and he ought to be fastidious in everything, for this is what the profession demands. He ought to have an appearance and approach that is distinguished. Everything ought to be in moderation, for these things are advantageous, so it is said. Be solicitous in your approach to the patient, not with head thrown back (arrogantly) or hesitantly with lowered glance, but with head inclined slightly as the art demands. He ought to hold his head humbly and evenly; his hair should not be too much smoothed down, nor his beard curled like that of a degenerate youth. He should approach the patient with moderate steps, not noisily, gazing calmly at the sick bed. He should endure peacefully the insults of the patients since those suffering from melancholic or frenetic ailments are likely to hurl evil words at physicians* [2]. Physicians' manners, dress, bearing, deportment, and conduct were vital and necessary elements of patient care, a tradition that extended from the earliest shamans to the emergence of scientific

B. Silverman, *The Power of Bedside Manners in Patient Care*,
https://doi.org/10.1007/978-3-032-10496-0_10

medicine. The Hippocratic corpus has many references to appropriate conduct and medical etiquette, with several devoted just to physician behavior (Figs. 10.1, 10.2 and 10.3).

In medieval Europe Physicians were usually clergy or scholars. They wore long robes and academic gowns, signaling education and social status rather than hygiene. With the enlightenment doctors increasingly dressed like scholars: black robes, stiff collars, sometimes wigs (mirroring other learned professions). The physician's authority was tied to learning, so dress was meant to reflect dignity and intellect rather than cleanliness. With the advances in science in the nineteenth century, especially with advances in microbiology, medicine began emphasizing cleanliness. In the mid-to-late 1800s, surgeons began wearing aprons and dark clothing—which often became bloodstained, ironically seen as a mark of experience. By the late 1800s, sterile technique was introduced, and white coats began to appear in laboratories and gradually in hospitals, symbolizing purity and science. By the early 1900s, the white coat became the universal symbol of physicians, replacing black scholarly robes. It represented scientific rigor, sterility, and authority. Stethoscopes, introduced in the early nineteenth century, became common accessories by the 20th, reinforcing the physician's image. In the mid-1900s professional dress also included tie, dress shirt, and conservative skirt/dress for women physicians. As infection control and comfort gained importance, scrubs—once confined to the operating room—spread to other hospital areas. Long white coats remained common for attendings and academic physicians, but residents, medical students, and ED/ICU staff increasingly wore scrubs. Now in the twenty-first century the white coat still signals professionalism, but scrubs are the standard dress

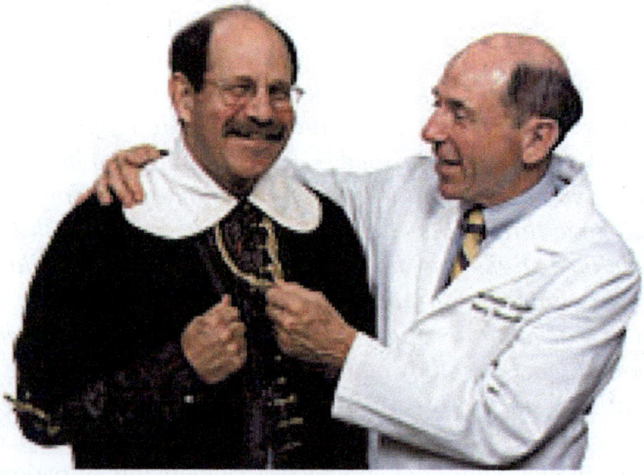

Fig. 10.1 The history of physician dress is fascinating—it reflects not only changes in fashion, but also evolving ideas about medicine, professionalism, hygiene, and authority. My brother addressed the Emory School of Medicine Anatomy class in the dress of William Harvey in 1628 when he described the circulation of the blood. I have my arm around him wearing the classic physician's attire of 1990

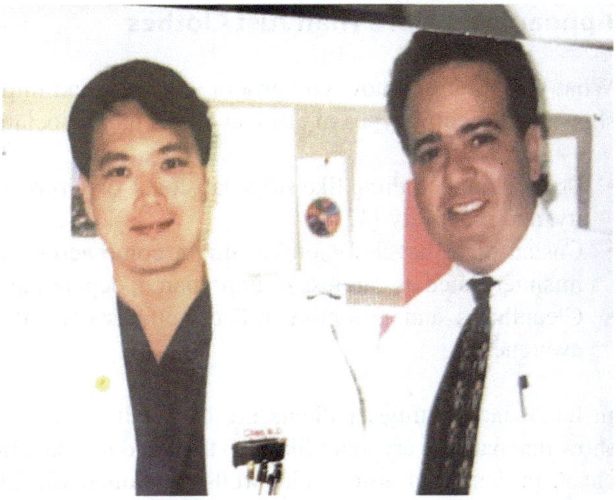

Fig. 10.2 My colleagues in the usual dress for 2000 when scrubs were becoming the standard in the hospital but a tie or dress was worn in the office

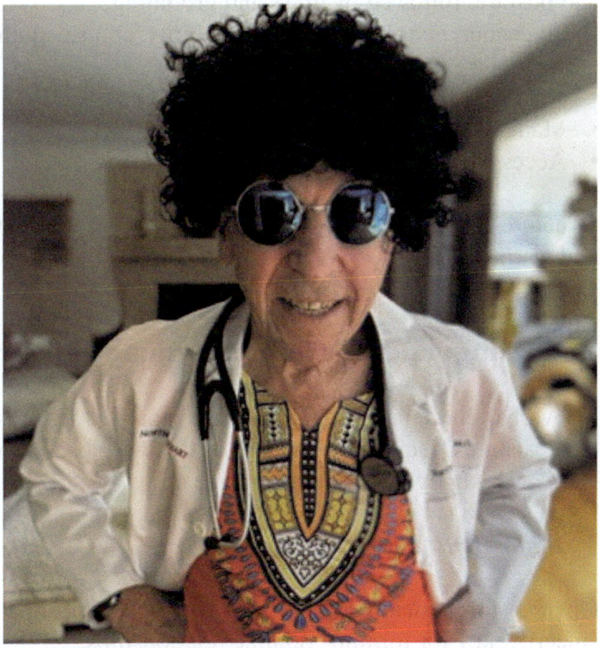

Fig. 10.3 This outfit and appearance are unlikely to encourage patient trust and confidence

even in the office setting but definitely in the hospital, OR, and ED. The stethoscope is a necklace worn more as a sign of stature than as a diagnostic tool. Business causal often without a white coat is increasing popular especially in the office, with telemedicine and on hospital rounds.

Appearance: More Than Just Clothes

What you wear and how you groom yourself send immediate signals. Psychology shows that specific types of attire evoke strong associations [3]:

- Professional clothing like suits, lab coats, or scrubs suggest competence, authority, and reliability [4].
- Casual or disheveled clothing might come across as relaxed—but can also be misinterpreted as careless or unprepared, depending on context.
- Cleanliness and grooming reflect self-respect, attention to detail, and social awareness.

In healthcare settings, patients are especially influenced by visual cues. Studies show that patients are more likely to trust and feel satisfied with providers who wear clean, professional attire—like well-maintained white coats or tidy scrubs. These visual impressions are formed in milliseconds, beginning with facial expressions and posture, followed by dress and grooming.

To encourage trust and approachability, choose clothing that is:

- Neat, well-fitted, and neutral in tone
- Made of soft, comfortable fabrics
- Accessorized simply and tastefully

Structured yet approachable outfits often strike the best balance between authority and warmth.

Body Language: The Silent Language of Connection

Nonverbal communication often says more than words. In patient care, your posture, gestures, facial expressions, and use of space can build—or break—rapport. Here's why body language is so critical:

1. ***Builds Trust and Connection***

Open gestures, steady eye contact, and relaxed posture foster a sense of safety and sincerity, key for forming genuine relationships.

2. ***Supports What You Say***

Nods, smiles, and leaning slightly forward show you're listening and engaged. These subtle cues reinforce your words and demonstrate empathy.

3. ***Reveals Emotions***

Facial expressions and body posture often communicate feelings more clearly than speech. People quickly sense disinterest, discomfort, or warmth based on your demeanor.

4. ***Respects Boundaries***

Personal space matters. Too much distance feels cold; too little feels invasive. Appropriate use of touch (like a handshake or reassuring hand on the arm) can comfort—when culturally and situationally appropriate.

5. ***Avoids "Computer-First" Interactions***

Never let a screen come between you and the patient. Patients feel disconnected when you focus more on your computer than on them. Instead, include the computer as a tool in the conversation—**not the center of it**.

A Tale of Two Encounters

Imagine this:

- A provider maintains warm eye contact, sits with an open posture, leans slightly forward, and reacts naturally as the patient speaks.
- Another provider avoids eye contact, crosses their arms, frequently checks their computer or phone, and leans back.

Both may use polite words—but the first will almost certainly leave a stronger, more positive impression. The second may unintentionally seem distracted, disinterested, or even untrustworthy.

Practical Body Language Tips for Patient Care

Keep these in mind to enhance communication and connection:

1. **Maintain Comfortable Eye Contact**
    - Look at the patient while speaking, with natural pauses.
    - Shows confidence and attentiveness.
2. **Smile Genuinely**
    - Especially when greeting, expressing empathy, or acknowledging patient emotions.
    - A warm smile creates a sense of safety and approachability.

3. **Adopt an Open Posture**
   - Avoid crossed arms or tightly crossed legs.
   - Keep shoulders relaxed, body facing the patient, and lean in slightly.
4. **Use Mirroring**
   - Subtly match the patient's gestures or posture to build subconscious rapport.
5. **Keep Hands Visible and Purposeful**
   - Use hand gestures naturally.
   - Avoid fidgeting, touching your face, or hiding your hands.
6. **Match Your Voice to the Moment**
   - Use a warm, steady tone.
   - Speak clearly and at a moderate pace—avoid monotone delivery.
7. **Practice Active Listening**
   - Nod occasionally, give verbal cues like "I see" or "That makes sense."
   - Avoid looking at screens or distractions.
8. **Face the Patient Directly**
   - Position yourself so no barriers—especially a computer—interfere with the interaction.

The Computer in the Exam Room: Balancing Technology and Human Connection

The computer has become a ubiquitous part of modern medical practice. It is now required for documenting every patient encounter, from the initial history and physical to the review of systems, physical exam findings, and the assessment and plan. Physicians must also record problem lists, lab results, medications, and other essential details within the electronic medical record (EMR).

While this documentation is critical for continuity of care, billing, and legal purposes, the computer has also emerged as a major source of stress and burnout for physicians. More importantly, it can interfere with the most vital element of medical practice: a meaningful doctor–patient relationship.

Navigating the "Triangle" of Physician, Patient, and Computer

During a patient encounter, the physician is inevitably managing two interactions at once—one with the patient and one with the computer. If the computer dominates, the physician may appear distracted or disengaged, leading patients to feel unheard or reduced to data points. Conversely, when the patient is prioritized and the computer minimized, the encounter regains its human connection.

Practical strategies can help strike this balance:

- **Room setup matters.** Position the computer so it does not physically block your view of the patient. Ideally, you should be able to maintain eye contact and an open posture during conversation.

- **Transparency builds trust.** Acknowledge your use of the computer during the visit: "*Let me take a moment to enter this information so we have a complete and accurate record.*"
- **Invite patient participation.** Frame the computer as a shared tool rather than a barrier. For example: "*I'm adding this problem to your list and noting our plan—this way, you'll be able to see it on your patient portal.*"

By explaining what you are doing, you reinforce the idea that documentation is part of the patient's care—not a distraction from it.

Balancing Attention Between Patient and Chart

There are times when full concentration on the computer is necessary, particularly when documenting complex histories, medication lists, or test results. In these moments, it is appropriate to let the patient know:

> *I need just a minute to carefully record this so we have all the details correct.*

This brief explanation reassures the patient that the physician is not simply "ignoring" them but is ensuring accuracy in their medical record.

Turning a Challenge into an Opportunity

The presence of the computer in the exam room is not inherently negative. When used thoughtfully, it can actually strengthen the physician–patient relationship. By sharing the screen, reviewing results together, and involving patients in building their care plan, the physician can transform the computer into a tool of collaboration and transparency.

Ultimately, the goal is to make the computer serve the patient, not overshadow them. With conscious effort, physicians can preserve the intimacy of the clinical encounter while still meeting the demands of modern documentation.

In Summary

Your appearance and body language are essential tools in building trust, respect, and effective communication. In healthcare, where human connection matters deeply, these subtle elements shape the entire patient experience. Present yourself with intention—you're not just treating a condition; you're connecting with a person.

The following images are visual examples for you to consider when presenting yourself to your patients. Consider the facial expressions, body language, style of your hair, facial hair, the type of outfit, how the clothes fit, are you engaging with your patient? All of these and more influence your patient's attitude about your interest and concern for their wellbeing. Study them and make your own judgements about how you should dress and present yourself to your patients (Fig. 10.4, 10.5, 10.6, 10.7, 10.8, 10.9, and 10.10).

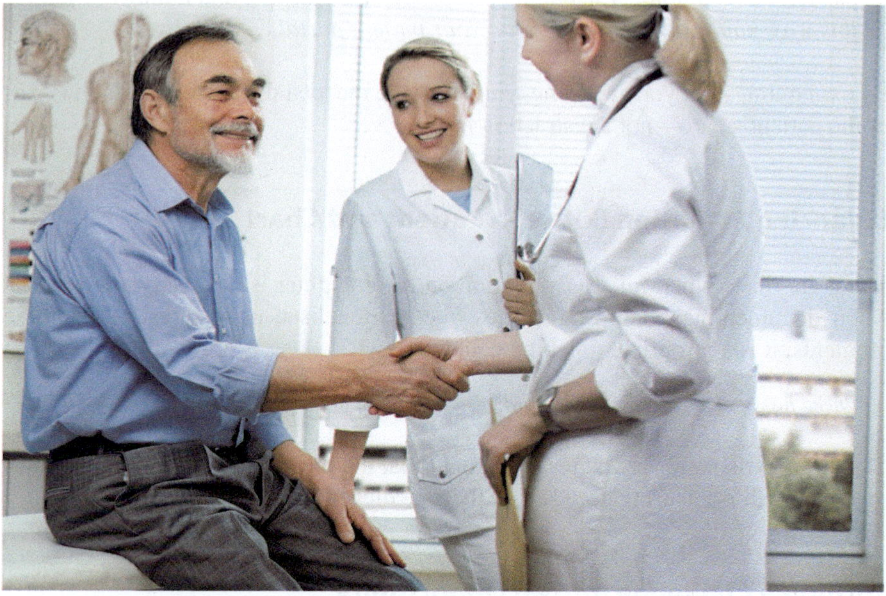

Fig. 10.4 The physician introducing herself to her patient. Her posture, eye contact, and handshake clearly demonstrate an interest in the patient as a person

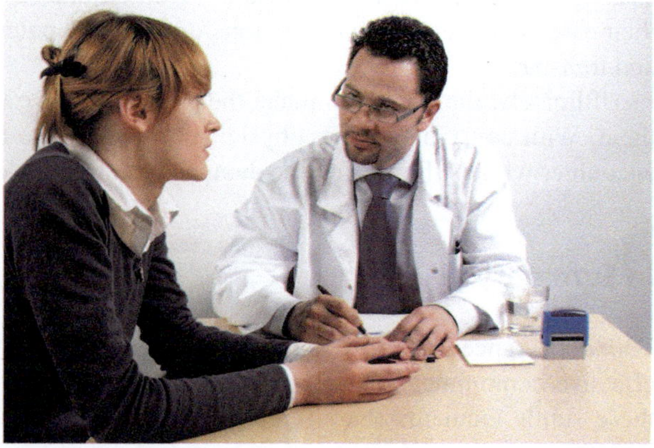

Fig. 10.5 A professionally dressed physician completely engaged with the patient, eye contact, body posture, and taking notes concerning the interview

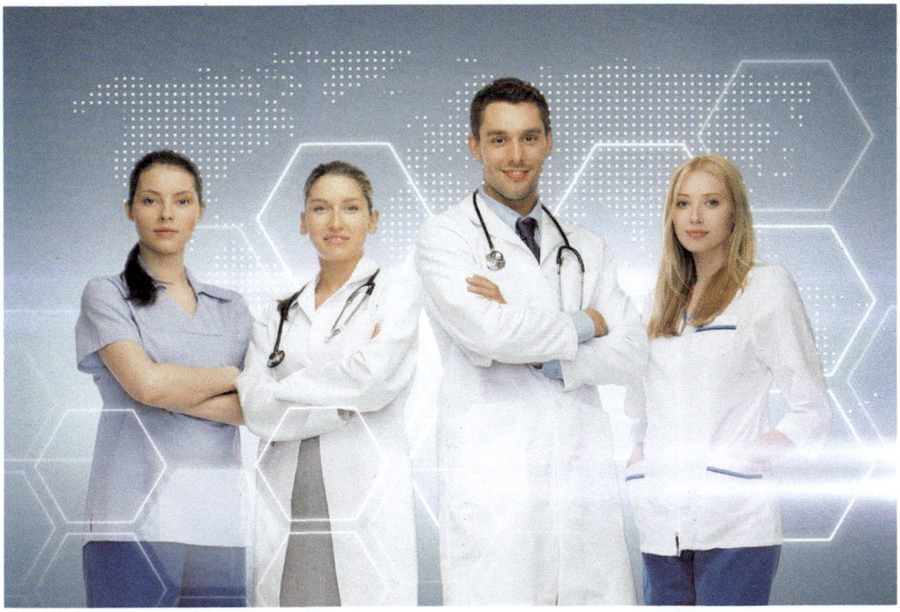

Fig. 10.6 Medical professionals all of them but their dress clearly identifies the physicians

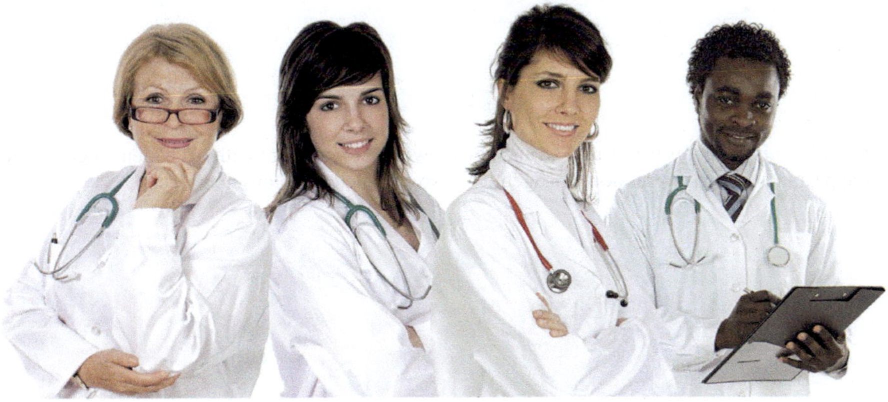

Fig. 10.7 Medical Students
How would you judge their appearance?
What are the features that foster confidence and trust?

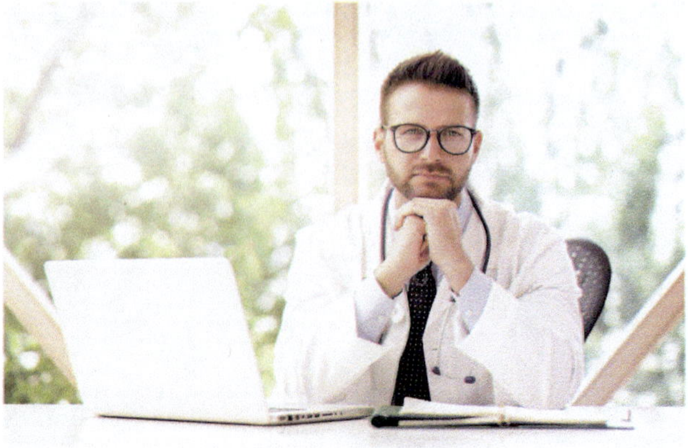

Fig. 10.8 Our Nemesis is the computer!
Do not ever let it get between you and your patient

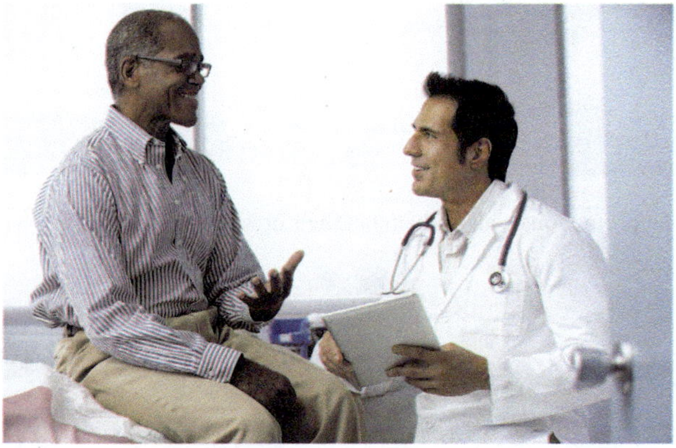

Fig. 10.9 This patient is using an iPad and not allowing it to interfere with his patient engagement
His appearance, facial expression, engagement is so complete and conscientious

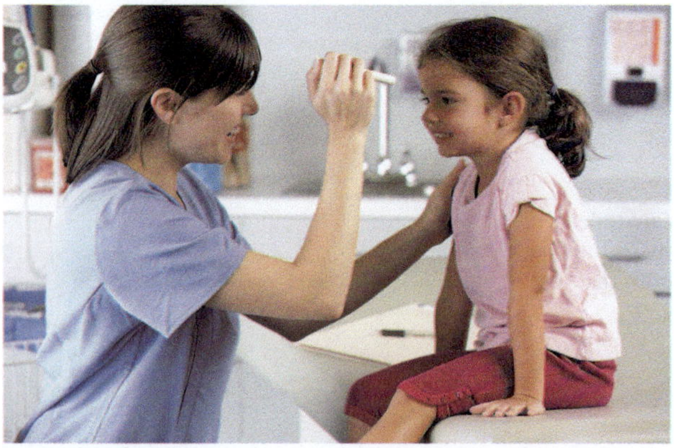

Fig. 10.10 Working with children is always a special challenge. The physician has engaged in a way to relax and reassure this child
This makes a frightening experience a happy and pleasant one

References

1. Zebrowitz LA, Montepare JM. Social psychological face perception: why appearance matters? Soc Personal Psychol Compass. 2008;2:1497–517. https://doi.org/10.1111/j.1751-9004.2008.00109.x.
2. Anonymous. Admonitions of Hippocrates of learning the history of medicine. In: Carmichael AG, Ratzan RM, editors. Medicine: a treasury of art and literature. New York: Hugh Lauter Levin Associates; 1991. p. 53–4.
3. Lennon SJ, Miller FG. Attire, physical appearance and first impressions: more is less. Clothing Textiles Res J. 1984–85;3:1–8.
4. Petrilli CM, Mack M, Petrilli JJ, Hickner A, Saint S, Chopra V. Understanding the role of physician attire on patient perceptions: a systematic review of the literature—targeting attire to improve likelihood of rapport (TAILOR) investigators. BMJ Open. 2015;5:e006578. https://doi.org/10.1136/bmjopen-2014-006578.

Recognizing and Responding to Bullying, Bias, and Harassment

11

Injustice anywhere is a threat to justice everywhere. (Martin Luther King Jr.)

Why Should You Be Concerned?

Bullying, harassment, and abuse are pervasive and serious issues in medicine [1]. It's crucial to recognize that none of us is immune. Recent data paints a troubling picture: 52% of female and 5% of male medical school faculty report experiencing sexual harassment. Additionally, over 20% of underrepresented minority medical students—compared to less than 4% of white students—report discrimination based on race or ethnicity. It is essential to identify such behavior when it occurs and to stand up against it (Fig. 11.1).

In 1982, pediatrician Dr. Henry Silver expressed concern about the mistreatment of medical students. He observed that students, once enthusiastic about their training, often emerged from it cynical and depressed, symptoms he had seen in abused or neglected children. This led him to question whether abuse and mistreatment could be contributing to these changes in medical students. In 1990, Dr. Silver published a survey that defined abuse as "to treat in a harmful, injurious, or offensive way; to attack in words; to speak insultingly, harshly, and unjustly to or about a person." His findings were shocking: 46% of first-year medical students reported experiencing abuse, and by the time students reached their fourth year, 80% had encountered some form of mistreatment. The highest incidence of abuse was reported during the first clinical year.

Sadly, Dr. Silver's concerns have not dissipated over time. In a 2019 survey by the Association of American Medical Colleges (AAMC), 40.4% of medical students reported some form of mistreatment during their training. Female and

B. Silverman, *The Power of Bedside Manners in Patient Care*,
https://doi.org/10.1007/978-3-032-10496-0_11

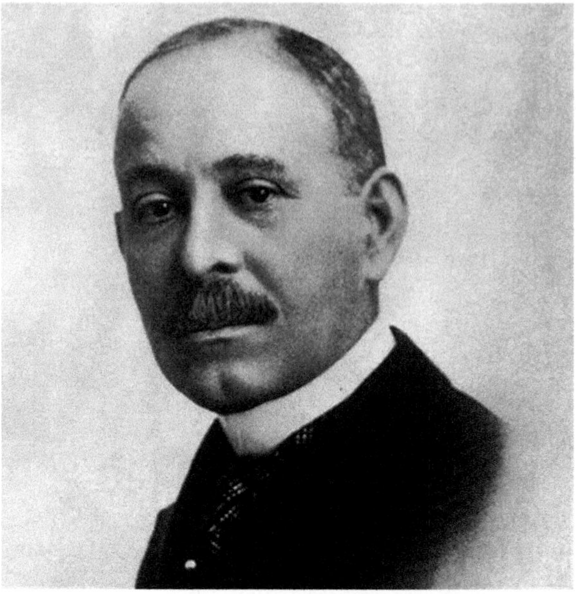

Fig. 11.1 Daniel Hale Williams Welcome CollectionHe was a pioneering Black physician born in 1856 in Pennsylvania. Williams apprenticed with a surgeon and trained at Chicago Medical College. He started a practice as one of only three Black physicians in the city and was able to teach anatomy at his Alma Mater but was denied hospital admitting privileges because of his race. In 1891, he founded Provident Hospital, the nation's first integrated training hospital for interns and nurses. In 1913, he was elected as the only Black charter member of the American College of Surgeons

non-white students were disproportionately affected. Other studies show that nearly 60% of students report experiences of harassment or discrimination, with verbal abuse being the most common and physical harassment affecting around 15% of students.

Defining Bullying and Harassment

The U.S. Equal Employment Opportunity Commission (EEOC) defines harassment as "unwelcome conduct based on race, color, religion, sex (including pregnancy), national origin, age (40 or older), disability, or genetic information." Harassment becomes unlawful when:

1. **Enduring the offensive conduct becomes a condition of continued employment.**
2. **The conduct is severe or pervasive enough to create a work environment that a reasonable person would consider intimidating or hostile.** [EEOC harassment]

In 2020, the U.S. Supreme Court expanded the definition of "sex" as a protected category to include gay, lesbian, and transgender workers. Federal protections apply to discrimination and harassment within the categories outlined above, but state laws and institutional policies may extend to other forms of discrimination or misconduct. Not all "unwelcome conduct" rises to the level of unlawful harassment, but repeated, systematic negative treatment—particularly in work or educational settings—can have damaging effects on individuals, resulting in stigmatization, psychological harm, and a loss of confidence and productivity.

Bullying in medicine is not limited to student-teacher dynamics. Patients and their families can also display racist or bullying behavior. In such difficult interactions, it's essential to listen to patient concerns while refusing to validate bias, hatred, or discrimination. Standing firm against inappropriate behavior—whether from a colleague, a superior, or a patient—helps maintain a culture of respect and accountability.

Responding to Bias, Discrimination, and Harassment [2]

The hierarchical nature of medical training makes students and residents particularly vulnerable to mistreatment [3]. They are often the least experienced members of the team, more prone to error, unfamiliar with established routines, and at the bottom of the power structure. This power imbalance can prevent individuals from speaking out. A student who feels uncomfortable with a comment from a professor may worry that speaking up will hurt her grades. A resident may fear retaliation when reporting mistreatment to a program director, potentially jeopardizing future opportunities. It's essential that trainees understand how to respond to and report bullying or harassment in a way that minimizes risk and ensures their voices are heard.

Assessing Bias

Over the past several years, there has been a growing recognition of the importance of addressing "implicit" or "unconscious" biases—attitudes or stereotypes that exist outside our conscious awareness but can still influence our interactions and decisions. According to the AAMC, "implicit biases are automatic associations—both positive and negative—that affect our understanding of, and actions toward, others based on characteristics like race, ethnicity, gender, age, and appearance." Research has shown that these biases can impact our behavior, even when we don't intend to be discriminatory.

Understanding that good intentions do not always protect us from acting on implicit biases is key. It's vital to challenge inappropriate comments or behaviors without attacking the person behind them. Criticizing an action rather than the individual can be far more effective in confronting problematic behavior. When you witness harassment or discrimination, it's important to have a strategy for speaking up. Silence allows harmful behavior to continue unchecked.

This call to action is a form of *active allyship*—a commitment to not only support those who are directly targeted but also to encourage others nearby to speak up and address the situation. The goal is to avoid normalizing toxic environments and instead foster a culture where respect and civility prevail. Challenging offensive comments requires courage, but responding with civility can create lasting change.

Key Takeaways

- Bullying and harassment are pervasive issues in medicine, disproportionately affecting women, people of color, and trainees.
- Understanding and recognizing what constitutes bullying and harassment is essential for addressing these behaviors.
- Having a strategy to respond to bullying and harassment helps prevent complicity through silence.
- Knowledge of institutional reporting systems is vital for safely addressing hate and harassment in the workplace or educational setting

References

1. Robertson JJ, Long B. Medicine's shame problem. Emerg Med. 2019;57:329–38. https://doi.org/10.1016/j.jemermed.2019.06.034.
2. Bromberg GK, Berwick JR, Horick NK, Burnett-Bowie SM. Experiences of bias in a multidisciplinary hospital medicine group. J Am Assoc Nurse Pract. 2024. https://doi.org/10.1097/JXX.0000000000000991.
3. Álvarez Villalobos NA, De León Gutiérrez H, Ruiz Hernandez FG, Elizondo Omaña GG, Vaquera Alfaro HA, Carranza Guzmán FJ. Prevalence and associated factors of bullying in medical residents: a systematic review and meta-analysis. J Occup Health. 2023;65:e12418. https://doi.org/10.1002/1348-9585.12418.

Managing the Electronic Medical Record, Social Media, and Technology in Medicine

12

Where Is the Computer When You're with the Patient?

First impressions begin the moment a patient walks through the door. Every interaction—with front-desk staff, nurses, and especially you, the physician—shapes their perception of your professionalism, empathy, and competence. Patients evaluate you through more than just your words. Body language, eye contact, tone of voice, and attentiveness all matter. The electronic medical record (EMR), while essential, should never interfere with that connection (Fig. 12.1).

Key Rule: **Never let the computer come between you and your patient.**

Position it to the side, so you can reference charts and enter data while maintaining open, direct communication. The patient—not the screen—should always be the focal point.

Evans RS. Electronic health records: then, now, and in the future. Yearb Med Inform. 2016;Suppl 1(Suppl 1):S48–61. https://doi.org/10.15265/IYS-2016-s006. PMID: 27199197; PMCID: PMC5171496.

B. Silverman, *The Power of Bedside Manners in Patient Care*, https://doi.org/10.1007/978-3-032-10496-0_12

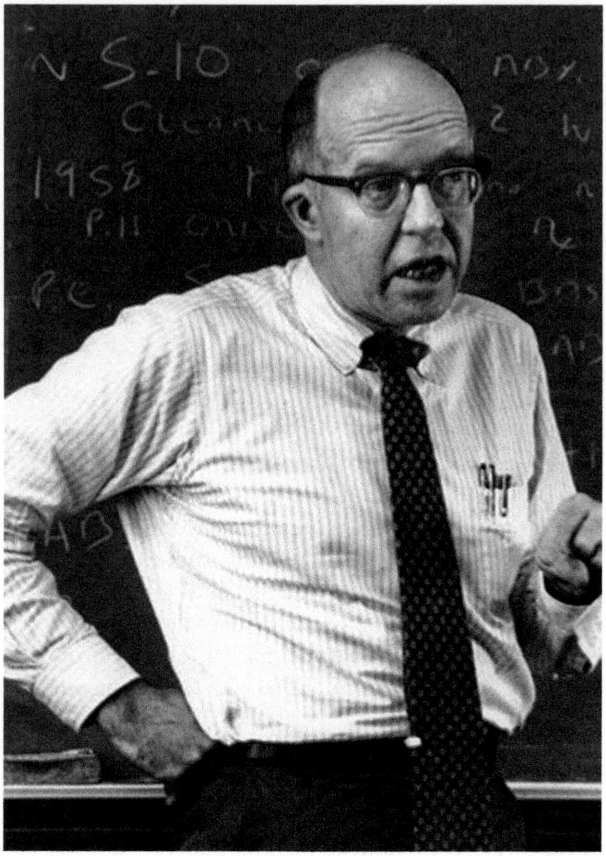

Fig. 12.1 Thomas Evans Brittingham. (Photo courtesy of Alan Graber)A legendary teacher on the medical wards at Vanderbilt Hospital. He felt one becomes a good physician by first learning how to effectively communicate. He taught that making and recording detailed and correct observations was essential in medicine

What Makes a Good Medical Progress Note?

A strong progress note is more than a routine entry—it's a tool for safe, effective, and coordinated care. The best notes are **clear, concise, accurate, and clinically useful**. They communicate the patient's current condition, your interpretation, and your plan, while also serving as a legal and billing document [1].

This isn't a step-by-step guide to writing SOAP notes, but rather a summary of the key qualities that make a progress note effective:

1. Use a Structured Format (SOAP or APSO)

   Most clinicians rely on SOAP (Subjective, Objective, Assessment, Plan) or APSO (Assessment, Plan, Subjective, Objective). Structure ensures clarity and efficiency.
   - **Subjective (S):** Patient's report of symptoms, concerns, or interval changes.
   - **Objective (O):** Vital signs, physical exam, labs, imaging, consult notes.

- **Assessment (A):** Your synthesis—differential diagnoses, trends, interpretation of data.
- **Plan (P):** Specific next steps for each problem—diagnostic, therapeutic, and follow-up.

2. Keep It Focused
   - Avoid re-documenting the entire H&P every day.
   - Highlight **interval changes** since the last note
   - Summarize **trends** (e.g., "Creatinine improved to 1.5 from 2.2 yesterday").
3. Organize by Problems
   - Frame the note around **active problems** (e.g., pneumonia, diabetes, hypertension).
   - For each: state current status → provide assessment → outline plan.
4. Write Clearly and Briefly
   - Use short, direct sentences.
   - Avoid vague terms or jargon.
   - Make your reasoning explicit so the next provider understands your thought process.
5. Make Plans Actionable
   - Recommendations should be **specific and practical** (e.g., "Continue ceftriaxone; switch to oral when afebrile for 48 h" instead of "Continue antibiotics").
   - Always include **next steps** (labs, imaging, consults, discharge planning).
6. Enhance Communication
   - Anticipate what colleagues (nurses, consultants, primary team) need to know to ensure continuity of care.
   - Document important conversations with the patient or family.
7. Meet Legal & Billing Standards
   - Include enough detail to justify the level of service (complexity, time, decision-making).
   - Avoid copying forward outdated information.
   - Write notes that can stand alone for audits, reviews, or legal purposes.

Example (SOAP-Style)

S: Patient reports improved breathing, no PND or orthopnea. Walking in neighborhood without symptoms

O: Afebrile, HR 68. BP 122/78 Lab BNP 100 CXR: pulmonary edema resolved

A: Heart Failure with reduced LV function improved and stable

P: Continue Coreg 25 mg BID, losartan 50 mg daily, dapagliflozin 10 mg qd, furosemide 40 mg qd, spironolactone 25 mg qd, follow exercise prescription, low sodium diet and periods of rest.

Using Digital Communication & Social Media in Medicine

Protect Patient Privacy Above All

- Never post identifiable patient information (names, faces, dates, unique cases) without explicit consent.
- Even "de-identified" details can sometimes be recognized—when in doubt, leave it out.
- Remember: HIPAA (in the U.S.) and similar laws elsewhere apply online just as they do in the hospital.

Maintain Professionalism

- Assume everything you post is **public and permanent**, even in private groups or "disappearing" messages.
- Hold yourself to the same standard online as you would in the exam room or lecture hall.
- Avoid posts that could be perceived as disrespectful, discriminatory, or unprofessional.

Separate Personal and Professional Identities

- Consider keeping professional accounts (for education, advocacy, or networking) distinct from personal ones.
- Be mindful of boundaries if patients try to connect with you on personal platforms.
- Check privacy settings regularly, but don't rely on them to protect you.

Communicate Responsibly

- Texting/email with patients: follow institutional policies and use secure, encrypted platforms when possible.
- Avoid giving specific medical advice on public platforms; instead, provide general health education and direct people to appropriate resources.
- Keep messages clear, respectful, and concise—remember they may be forwarded or saved.

Use Social Media Positively

- Share accurate health information to combat misinformation.
- Use it to advocate for public health, amplify evidence-based practices, and engage in professional education.
- Connect with colleagues, mentors, and professional organizations for learning and collaboration.

Know the Risks

- Be aware of legal, ethical, and reputational risks of online activity.
- A single unprofessional post can damage trust or credibility.
- Always pause and ask: *Would I be comfortable if this post appeared on the front page of tomorrow's newspaper?*

Bottom Line
Use digital communication and social media as tools for **education, advocacy, and professional connection**, but always with **privacy, professionalism, and caution** in mind.

Digital Communication & Social Media in Medicine

Top 10 Do's and Don'ts for Students & Residents

Do's

1. **Protect Patient Privacy**
   – De-identify all patient details; when in doubt, don't post.
2. **Stay Professional**
   – Assume everything online is public and permanent.
3. **Use Secure Channels**
   – Communicate via hospital-approved, encrypted platforms.
4. **Educate & Advocate**
   – Share evidence-based health info, fight misinformation.
5. **Build Your Professional Identity**
   – Use social media to connect with mentors, peers, and medical communities.

Don't

6. **Don't Post Patient Info**
   – Even "anonymized" stories may be recognizable.
7. **Don't Cross Boundaries**
   – Avoid friending/following patients on personal accounts.
8. **Don't Share Unverified Info**
   – Posting inaccurate health info can harm patients and credibility.
9. **Don't Vent Publicly**
   – Complaints about patients, colleagues, or institutions can be damaging.
10. **Don't Forget Your Digital Footprint**
    – Every post can follow you throughout your career.

Quick Check Before You Post:

Would I be comfortable if this were on the front page of tomorrow's paper—or shown to my attending?

Key Takeaways

1. **Be Professional Online**
   Use social platforms to share knowledge, not clinical care.

2. **Respect Privacy**
   Never share patient information—ever.
3. **Avoid Venting Publicly**
   Don't post in frustration about colleagues, institutions, or patients.
4. **Offer Constructive Communication**
   Thoughtful criticism and advice are fine when done respectfully and in the right forum.
5. **Think Before You Engage**
6. When in doubt, leave it out

Bottom Line Your words—online and in person—carry weight. Stay professional. Stay respectful. And always put the patient first, whether you're face-to-face or communicating through a screen.

Reference

1. Schrager S. Writing clinical notes: have we made progress? Fam Pract Manag. 2022;29(4):3–4.

13 Essential Bedside Behaviors for the Care of Hospitalized Patients

The patient is neither a disease to be discussed, nor a showcase of pathologic interest, nor a dispassionate bystander. He is a sick person in the alien environment of the hospital, disturbed by his illness and involved in it at least as much as the doctors. He is anxious to know what is happening, entitled to find out, and generally able to make helpful contributions to all aspects of his clinical management. (Alvan Feinstein [1])

The Hospital: A Sacred Yet Complex Place of Care

The hospital is a place of dualities—a revered sanctuary of medicine and technology, yet also a high-risk environment where patients can succumb to disease, hospital-acquired infections, or accidents. Despite these hazards, most leave in better health, some cured, others on the road to recovery, often amazed by the tender, empathetic care they receive. Medical science has made leaps in diagnosis, treatment, and technology. We have seen tremendous changes in the hospital environment with nurses no longer dressed in starched white uniforms, and doctors' suits and ties replaced with scrubs. Medical records are now instantly accessible, and many new diagnostic tools are available at our fingertips. But have these advances improved the way we interact with patients? Do we still place the patient's well-being at the center of care, or have we become too focused on the technicalities of medicine? Sir Robert Platt, a professor of medicine, warned that clinical science risks neglecting the emotional and irrational aspects of human behavior in health and disease. He emphasized that the basic facts of happiness and unhappiness in a patient's life are just as important as biochemistry and physiology (Fig. 13.1).

B. Silverman, *The Power of Bedside Manners in Patient Care*,
https://doi.org/10.1007/978-3-032-10496-0_13

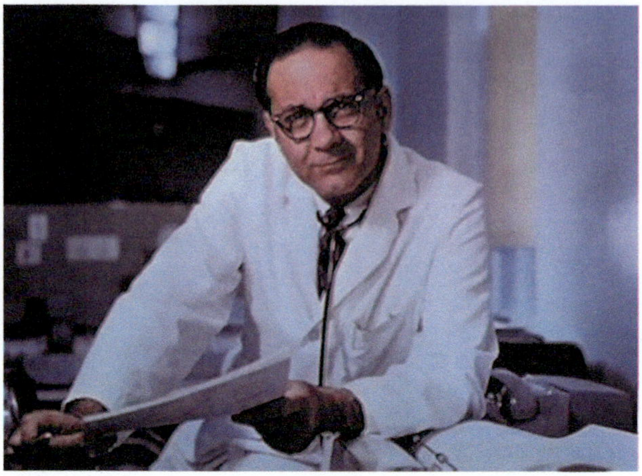

Fig. 13.1 Alvan R. Feinstein Wellcome Collection

The Hospitalized Patient Is a Special Concern

The hospital setting is often fraught with anxiety and distress. Patients and their families face a range of physical discomforts and emotional challenges—uncomfortable waiting rooms, uncertainty about test results, and the discomfort of fasting before procedures. A dismissive admitting clerk, a brusque nurse, or an unengaged doctor can make the environment feel even more threatening, turning patients into mere numbers in a system. Healthcare should be about healing, not just diagnosis and treatment. The human touch—rooted in empathy, kindness, and respect—is often what sets excellent care apart from good care. William Stokes of the famous nineteenth century Dublin School of Medicine commented on the influence of the hospital wards on medical practice; *In the wards of the hospital the student learns that which cannot be taught in the dissecting room or in the theatre; he learns to teach himself to act and discover. And he does much more. The kindlier feeling of his heart is stirred, and he becomes so trained to works of charity and mercy that their practice is at last a second nature. He acquires that moral courage by which at the call of duty, or of mercy which is duty he learns to despise danger, and to meet death whether it comes by pestilence or by the sword* [2].

Emergency Department: A Delicate Balance of Compassion and Efficiency

The emergency department (ED) is the beating heart of the hospital—a microcosm of organized chaos, where every team member plays a critical role in the patient's outcome. The physician is often seen as the leader of the team. In the fast-paced ED, efficiency is essential, but it's important to recognize and serve the patient's immediate needs. This means keeping the patient informed as to the status of their evaluation, checking on their wellbeing at least every 15–20 minutes, informing them of why there are delays and whether there is information when they will have an answer or treatment.

The ED is where many patients first encounter the hospital, often in a state of distress. Physicians must balance the need for swift, accurate diagnosis with the emotional needs of their patients, who may be anxious, scared, or in pain. It's essential that patients feel heard and respected, especially when they are vulnerable. Small gestures—such as providing estimated wait times, regularly checking in with patients, and offering reassurance—can have a significant impact on patient satisfaction and outcomes. This requires not only medical skill but also compassion and empathy. The goal is not just to diagnose and treat, but to ease the patient's suffering in the process.

The Cost of Caring

While medical advances have greatly improved patient care, the costs of these advancements have risen exponentially. An ED visit, once affordable, is now a significant financial burden for many, even for those with insurance. It is crucial that healthcare providers remain mindful of the cost of care and strive to use resources judiciously. Remember order only those studies necessary for diagnosing the complaint which brought the patient to the ED.

Putting Patients First

At the end of the day, patient care is about more than just accurate diagnoses and treatments; it's about the patient's overall experience. This includes ensuring their comfort, addressing their emotional needs, and navigating the complexities of the healthcare system in a way that minimizes their stress and suffering. In a healthcare environment that often feels impersonal, it's important to remember the profound impact that thoughtful, compassionate care can have on a patient's recovery. From reducing wait times to improving communication, every interaction—no matter how small—can make a difference in a patient's journey through the hospital.

The Hospital Inpatient Service: A Dynamic Environment for Care

Working in a hospital differs significantly from a typical outpatient office. While a well-run office often involves routine cases with a small team, the hospital is a high-stakes, fast-paced environment. The complexity of care increases dramatically as patients require inpatient services. For many physicians, the most intense and exciting moments in medicine happen in the hospital, particularly in the OR and ICU. In this environment, effective communication is key. You'll interact with a wide range of professionals: nurses, physical therapists, pharmacists, social workers, radiologists, and administrative staff. Each plays a critical role in patient care, and it's essential to treat everyone with respect and appreciation. This fosters a collaborative atmosphere and leads to better patient outcomes.

The Role of Nursing in Inpatient Care

Nurses are at the heart of hospital care. Physicians spend less time with patients, nurses are present 24/7, monitoring progress, addressing concerns, and engaging with families. Effective communication between physicians and nurses is crucial, and it's important to respect their expertise. When rounding, make sure to read the nurse's notes and, if necessary, leave a message for them to call you when they're free. Engaging nurses in patient discussions can provide valuable insights. If issues arise with nursing care, address them privately with the charge nurse—never in front of patients or staff.

Communication on the Hospital Floor

Effective communication is vital for quality patient care, and there are **four main methods of communication in the hospital**: direct person-to-person interaction, written notes (especially in the EMR), texting or emailing, and telephone calls. Each method has its own rules of etiquette.

Direct Communication Person-to-person interaction is the most effective form of communication, allowing for clear exchange of ideas. It's essential to communicate directly with colleagues, especially in emergencies. For non-urgent matters, leave a message with time windows for a return call. Avoid interrupting others unnecessarily but ensure that important patient-related calls are returned promptly.

Progress Notes Well-written progress notes are critical for coordinating patient care. In the past, handwritten notes were often illegible and incomplete, but the introduction of electronic medical records (EMRs) has improved legibility. However, many EMR notes still suffer from being overly detailed, making it hard to extract useful information. A good progress note should be:

- **Meaningful**: Focus on current symptoms and findings, without repeating excessive historical data.
- **Decipherable**: Avoid clutter by only including relevant information from previous notes and tests.
- **Instructive**: Provide insights on patient progress, response to treatment, and upcoming care plans. Document interactions with family and start discharge planning early.

Texting This is a good way to let colleagues, nurses, and staff know you have received their information, read their notes, or completed a task like reviewing images. You can also let them know when you are available or will be on the wards. You can share your cell phone number and ask them to call you if that is necessary. You cannot share any personal patient information by a text.

Phone Calls This is an excellent way to communicate but because EVERYONE is busy. It is often helpful to text or leave a message at the nursing station to ask when is a good time for both of you to talk.

The Importance of Good Manners

In a hospital, every interaction—whether with patients, families, or staff—should be approached with kindness, respect, and professionalism. Small gestures of appreciation, like thanking housekeeping or acknowledging the efforts of nursing staff, go a long way in improving morale and ensuring everyone is working toward the same goal: providing the best care for patients. The hospital is a complex and dynamic environment where teamwork and effective communication are essential. Respect for all members of the healthcare team, from nurses to administrators is vital. This fosters better care for patients and a more positive working environment. By practicing good communication, professionalism, and empathy, you'll be better equipped to navigate the challenges and rewards of inpatient care.

Who Is in Charge?

In the hospital, the hospitalist physician oversees the patient. Most patients will have several physicians involved in their care. In surgery this may include the surgeon, anesthesiologist, oncologist, and infectious disease physicians; in medicine the cardiologist, nephrologist, gastroenterologist, infectious diseases, or many other specialties including hospice care. The various individual organs or disease processes, each studied by separate specialties and considered individually, are complex parts of a whole entity, the patient. Every caregiver as well as the patient and the family must be sure there is open, clear communication among all the caregivers and patient and family. It is essential for good patient care.

Patients may be too ill, too confused, or too anxious to really understand what the physician is trying to communicate. Every time you talk with your patient consider their state of mind and judge how much information can be understood. You may need a family member present or ask the nurse to reinforce your instructions. Consider reviewing the discharge instructions over time such as daily for several days. Always provide detailed written information for the patient. It is necessary to:

1. Inform your patient and/or their family of the tests you are ordering.
2. Explain why you ordered the tests.
3. Tell them when they will receive the results.
4. Let the family know when you plan to round, and if that is not possible obtain a family contact number so you can share important information and answer questions.

The hospitalist is always in the hospital, so it is easier for the family to communicate with that physician. But remember, if the question concerns a surgical issue, the patient and family will want to hear directly from the surgeon. The same is true if the patient suffered a heart attack–they want to speak with the cardiologist. The hospitalist may be coordinating care, but the patient and family will want to hear from each physician caring for the patient.

Caring for the Patient

Abraham Verghese, a physician and best-selling author, in a 2011 TED talk on patient care, expresses concern that modern medicine is losing touch with the human connection of patient care. He felt electronic health records can negatively impact the patient-physician relationship by potentially reducing face-to-face time and leading to physician burnout. Patients and families can be lost in this system, and it is absolutely necessary to remember the focus of concern is caring for the whole patient as well as treating their disease. As Claude Bernard, the French physiologist who first used the "scientific method" said; "*A physician is by no means physician to living beings in general, not even physician to the human race, but rather, physician to a human individual in certain morbid conditions peculiar to himself and forming what is called his idiosyncrasy.*"

Dialogue with the Family

There is a group game in which the players create a picture or story. The first player draws a picture or tells a very brief story in secret to the next player. As the picture or story is passed around, considerable changes occur until by the time it reaches the originator of the story, the narrative or picture has changed considerably. Something similar happens when multiple physicians and PAs confer with patients and family from their different perspectives. When discussing prognosis, long term care, rehabilitation, and death one needs to be sure all are on the same page as the managing physician. It is always wise to discuss discharge planning directly with the managing physician and patient's nurse when the patient is close to discharge. Do not depend on the progress notes, nurse's comments, or social service alone. Some aspects of the care plan can only be properly managed if the lead physician is fully informed. A patient may become confused or even unnerved if multiple comments suggest multiple courses of action. It should be obvious that any advice concerning diet, lifestyle, medications, rehabilitation and follow-up must be written.

Addressing Abusive and Disruptive Behavior on the Ward

Sir William Osler once observed that the practice of medicine "among our fellow creatures is often a testy and choleric business." In other words, tensions can run high in clinical settings. Yet professionalism—grounded in good manners and mutual respect—is not merely a courtesy; it is a moral imperative.

The Joint Commission has established standards specifically addressing disruptive and inappropriate behavior in healthcare institutions, recognizing that such conduct can directly compromise patient safety and outcomes.

To maintain a positive clinical environment, avoid conflicts with colleagues, staff, and patients on the ward. When tensions arise, step away from the bedside and seek resolution in a private setting. Involving a neutral third party—such as a nursing supervisor, administrator, or trusted colleague—can help facilitate a constructive outcome.

Responsibilities to the Patient in the Emergency Department (ED)

1. **Keep the patient and family informed** at every stage of care.
2. **Clearly explain any tests** you order—what they are, why they are needed, and what they may reveal.
3. **Provide an estimated wait time** for test results to manage expectations.
4. **Keep the family updated** on the patient's condition and any changes in status.
5. **When ordering non-emergency tests**, especially if they are costly, discuss more affordable alternatives if appropriate.
6. **Communicate with the patient at least every 20 min** to provide a status update and maintain trust.
7. **If follow-up testing or an office visit is recommended**, inform the patient of its urgency, timing, and help arrange the appointment before discharge, if possible.
8. **If the patient is being admitted**, continue monitoring and reassessing at least every 30 min until transfer to the inpatient unit is complete.

Responsibilities to the Patient on the Ward

1. **Inform the patient and family about any tests** that are ordered, including their purpose and when to expect results.
2. **Provide a general time window for rounds** so the patient and family know when to expect an update.
3. **Regularly communicate updates** about the patient's progress and care plan.

4. **Maintain consistent communication** with the entire healthcare team, including nurses, consultants, social workers, and ancillary staff.
5. **Ensure alignment at discharge**—all team members should understand and agree on the care plan.
6. **Facilitate smooth transitions of care** by communicating clearly with outpatient providers and arranging necessary follow-up.
7. **Always model respectful and professional communication** with colleagues and staff.
8. **Assign clear responsibility:** One physician should be accountable for final decisions, executing orders, and updating the family.
9. **Zero tolerance for disruptive behavior:** Inappropriate conduct that undermines patient care or team collaboration is unacceptable.

References

1. Feinstein AR. Clinical judgement. Robert E. Kruger Publishing. 1967. ISBN 10: 0882751417 ISBN 13: 9780882751412.
2. Stokes W. The discourse was delivered at the Meath Hospital in 1861 and printed as a pamphlet under the title *Medical Education.*

14 The Vital Role of Humility in Medicine

> *His [the physician] thoughtful management of the total problems of the sick person makes mere treatment of a disease or a symptom seem woefully inadequate. He is inexhaustibly capable of infusing into his patient's insight, self-discipline, optimism and courage. Those he cannot make well he comforts. Versed in medical science, he also understands human nature and enjoys working with it. The things he works with are intellectual capacity, unconfined clinical experience, and the perceptive use of his eye, ears, hands, and heart.*
> (Phillip Tumulty The Johns Hopkins clinician)

In a bustling hospital, a seasoned physician pauses to consult a junior colleague about a puzzling diagnosis. This act—rooted in humility—exemplifies a core truth: medicine thrives not on infallibility but on the willingness to acknowledge limitations. Humility, often defined as the ability to recognize one's strengths and weaknesses without arrogance, is indispensable in healthcare. It fosters patient trust, enhances collaboration, drives lifelong learning, and mitigates errors, ultimately elevating the quality of care (Fig. 14.1).

B. Silverman, *The Power of Bedside Manners in Patient Care*,
https://doi.org/10.1007/978-3-032-10496-0_14

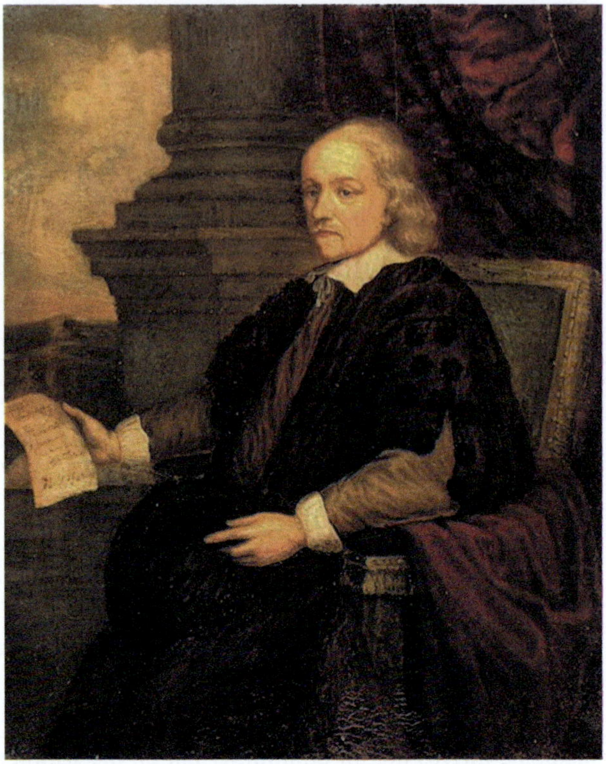

Fig. 14.1 William Harvey Wellcome CollectionDiscovered the circulation of blood and the heart's role as the pump, a discovery that revolutionized medical physiology. At the time of Harvey's discovery Galen's concepts dominated medical thinking. It was Harvey's outstanding character, his humility that allowed others to appreciate the importance of his discovery

Patient-Centered Care and Trust

Humility begins at the bedside. A humble clinician listens actively, valuing a patient's narrative as critical to diagnosis. Studies show that diagnostic errors often stem from inadequate patient engagement [1]. By prioritizing a patient's voice, physicians avoid biases and uncover subtle clues. Moreover, humility empowers patients, respecting their autonomy in shared decision-making. When a doctor admits uncertainty—such as explaining multiple treatment options—trust deepens, transforming the patient-provider relationship into a partnership rooted in transparency.

Collaboration in Healthcare Teams

Modern medicine relies on multidisciplinary teams, where humility dismantles hierarchical barriers. A surgeon humbly seeking an anesthesiologist's input or a nurse's observation exemplifies this. The 1999 Institute of Medicine report To Err Is Human highlighted communication failures as a leading cause of errors [2]. Humble teams foster psychological safety, enabling members to voice concerns without fear.

For example, during a complex surgery, a resident's hesitant question about a misplaced instrument might prevent a catastrophic oversight. Such collaboration, grounded in mutual respect, ensures comprehensive care.

Lifelong Learning

Medicine evolves rapidly; today's breakthroughs become obsolete tomorrow. Humility fuels the curiosity to learn, driving professionals to attend conferences, embrace new technologies, or seek mentorship. Consider the COVID-19 pandemic: clinicians worldwide humbly revised protocols as new data emerged. A physician's admission of knowledge gaps—whether about a novel therapy or cultural practices affecting care—prevents stagnation. This intellectual humility, as termed by psychologist Carol Dweck, cultivates a growth mindset essential for navigating medical advancements.

Error Prevention and Ethical Practice

Humility's most profound impact lies in error mitigation. Studies indicate that medical errors cause many deaths in the United States and many of these deaths are linked to overconfidence [3]. A humble practitioner openly reviews mistakes, engaging in root-cause analyses rather than concealing faults. Atul Gawande, in his book Complications, underscores how morbidity and mortality conferences normalize learning from errors. Ethically, humility aligns with the Hippocratic Oath's injunction to "do no harm," prioritizing patient welfare over ego.

Acknowledging Limits of Knowledge and Skills

Medicine is an ever-evolving field with new research, treatments, and technologies emerging regularly. Humility allows healthcare professionals to recognize that no one knows everything, and there is always more to learn. This recognition fosters continuous learning, encourages seeking second opinions when needed, and ensures that medical practitioners remain open to new ideas, clinical evidence, and evolving best practices.

Conclusion

Humility in medicine is not weakness but wisdom—a recognition that healing is a collective, ever-evolving endeavor. By embracing humility, clinicians strengthen patient relationships, enhance teamwork, pursue knowledge, and uphold ethical standards. In an era of advancing technology and complex care, humility remains the heartbeat of compassionate, effective medicine. Cultivating it institutionally through training and culture ensures healthcare systems not only cure but also connect, learn, and evolve. As Sir William Osler once commented, *in seeking for the truth you must be ever ready to admit that you may be wrong* [4]. He expressed *The greater the ignorance, the greater the dogmatism.* Humility bridges that distinction, reminding us that medicine, at its core, is human.

References

1. Stewart MA. Effective physician-patient communication and health outcomes: a review. CMAJ. 1995;152(9):1423–33. PMID: 7728691; PMCID: PMC1337906.
2. Institute of Medicine (US) Committee on Quality of Health Care in America. In: Kohn LT, Corrigan JM, Donaldson MS, editors. To err is human: building a safer health system. Washington, DC: National Academies Press; 2000.
3. Al-Maghrabi M, Mamade S, Schmidt HG, Omair A, Al-Nasser S, Alhari NS, Ali Magzoub MEM. Overconfidence, time-on-task, and medical errors: is there a relationship? Adv Med Educ Pract. 2024;15:133–40. https://doi.org/10.2147/AMEP.S442689.
4. Osler W. Aequanimitas 1889.

15 Divulging Sad News to Your Patient While Continuing to Provide Hope

What is your duty in the matter of telling a patient that he is probably the subject of an incurable disease? ... One thing is certain; it is not for you to don the black cap, and, assuming the judicial function, take hope from any patient—"hope that comes to all". (William Osler from Lectures on Angina Pectoris and Allied States)

The Power of Hope in Medicine

Hope is one of the most profound and powerful tools a physician can offer. At the bedside, even when a cure is out of reach, the physician's role is to provide hope—whether it's hope for healing, for comfort, or for dignity in the face of suffering [1].

In moments of fear, uncertainty, and despair, it is the physician who helps patients and families find light in the darkness. This requires more than clinical skill—it calls for emotional presence, empathy, and clear communication. When patients feel overwhelmed by illness, a lack of hope can easily spiral into despair. Compassionate, honest communication helps anchor patients, giving them the courage to confront whatever lies ahead—even when outcomes are uncertain (Fig. 15.1).

B. Silverman, *The Power of Bedside Manners in Patient Care*,
https://doi.org/10.1007/978-3-032-10496-0_15

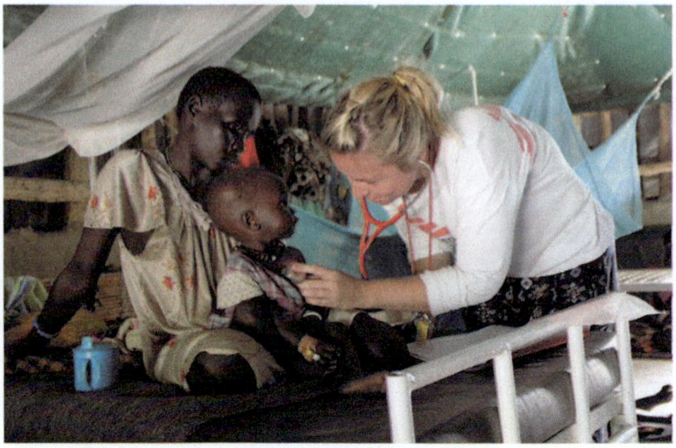

Fig. 15.1 Me'decins Sans Frontie'res**Doctors without Borders: Caring for the most Defenseless and Vulnerable**The organization has over 67,000 team members and is dedicated to the proposition that quality care matters and that developing countries deserve first rate medical care. A medical organization that brings hope to where there is often only despair

Communication as a Cornerstone of Care

Delivering difficult or life-altering news is one of the most delicate tasks a physician faces. It requires both precision and compassion. Missteps can lead to misunderstanding, misplaced hope, or even lasting resentment. That's why clear, empathetic communication is a core competency in medical training [2]. Physicians must avoid assumptions about what a patient feels or understands. Personal stories should be shared sparingly and only when truly helpful. Above all, language must be chosen with care—taking into account not only the medical facts but also the patient's cultural background and emotional readiness.

The Art of Delivering Difficult News

Breaking sad or life-changing news can be incredibly challenging—especially when there's little time to build rapport. In these moments, words like "cancer," "untreatable," or "ICU" can overwhelm, making it hard for patients to absorb anything that follows. The way information is delivered can profoundly affect how patients cope and respond. Even in the absence of a cure, hope can still be offered—through comfort, pain relief, and emotional presence.

Steps for Delivering Difficult News

1. **Set the Stage**: Create a private, quiet space. Silence your phone. Sit down to show that the patient has your full attention. A comforting gesture, like a light touch, can help build connection.

2. **Gauge Understanding**: Start with open-ended questions to assess what the patient knows and expects. Pay close attention to verbal and nonverbal cues.
3. **Deliver Information in Steps**: Use clear, simple language. Avoid jargon. Introduce bad news gently—never bluntly or without context.
4. **Respond with Empathy**: Acknowledge whatever the patient is feeling—shock, fear, sadness. Validate their emotions and let them know they're not alone.
5. **Offer a Clear Path Forward**: Whether it's a treatment plan or comfort-focused care, outline next steps clearly. Ask patients to repeat the plan to ensure understanding.
6. **Provide Ongoing Support**: Reassure the patient that you will remain a source of support. Compassion should never waver, regardless of the prognosis.

The SPIKES Protocol: A Structured Approach [3]

The **SPIKES** protocol offers a helpful, evidence-based framework for navigating these emotionally charged conversations:

- **S—Set up the interview**: Ensure privacy, dedicate uninterrupted time, and prepare mentally.
- **P—Perception**: Assess the patient's understanding of their condition.
- **I—Invitation**: Ask how much detail the patient wants to receive.
- **K—Knowledge**: Share information clearly, avoiding complex terminology.
- **E—Empathy**: Recognize and validate the patient's emotions.
- **S—Strategy and Summary**: Provide a plan, review next steps, and invite questions.

When Hope Doesn't Mean Cure

Even when recovery is no longer possible, there are still powerful forms of hope to offer. Hope can mean comfort. It can mean control over pain. It can mean the preservation of dignity or the presence of loved ones in a patient's final days. Hope, in its deepest sense, is about preserving a person's humanity. It's about helping patients feel heard, respected, and cared for. When medicine can no longer extend life, it can still enhance the quality of the time that remains.

Key Takeaways

1. **How should physicians deliver life-changing news?**
   - Create a private, safe space.
   - Understand the patient's perspective.
   - Use clear, compassionate language.

- Validate the patient's emotions.
- Present a clear, realistic plan.
- Offer continued emotional and physical support.

2. **What is the SPIKES Protocol?**

   A six-step approach for delivering difficult news:

- **S**et up the conversation
- Assess the patient's **P**erception
- Seek an **I**nvitation to share information
- Share **K**nowledge clearly
- Show **E**mpathy
- Create a **S**trategy for what comes next

3. **What can physicians offer when there's little chance of recovery?**

   They can offer relief from pain, respect for the patient's dignity, and emotional support. They can help the patient maintain agency and connection. Ultimately, they can offer the kind of hope that endures even when a cure is not possible.

In the end, hope is not just a feeling—it's an act of care. And sometimes, it is the most important medicine a doctor can give.

References

1. Velić S, Qama E, Diviani N, Rubinelli S. Patients' perception of hope in palliative care: a systematic review and narrative synthesis. Patient Educ Couns. 2023;115:107879. https://doi.org/10.1016/j.pec.2023.107879. Epub 2023 June 30. PMID: 37413808.
2. Fallowfield L, Jenkins V. Communicating sad, bad, and difficult news in medicine. Lancet. 2004;363(9405):312–9. https://doi.org/10.1016/S0140-6736(03)15392-5. PMID: 14751707.
3. Mahendiran M, Yeung H, Rossi S, Khosravani H, Perri GA. Evaluating the effectiveness of the SPIKES model to break bad news – a systematic review. Am J Hosp Palliat Care. 2023;40(11):1231–60. https://doi.org/10.1177/10499091221146296. Epub 2023 Feb 13. PMID: 36779374.

16 Building Trust with Children

Alone at the Bedside

The child lies small,
a hush of breath,
threads of life
pulled taut in her chest.

The parents hover—
their fear so raw
it nearly fills the room.
They look to him,
the one with answers,
the one who must not fail.

The doctor bends close,
not only to the child,
but to the impossible task:
to measure the distance
between what he knows
and what they need to hear.

He feels the gravity
in every silence,
each beat of the tiny heart
an unspoken demand
for vigilance, for certainty
no mortal can give.

His hands are steady
because they must be;
his voice quiet
because it cannot break.
The weight is his alone—
to guard the child,

B. Silverman, *The Power of Bedside Manners in Patient Care*,
https://doi.org/10.1007/978-3-032-10496-0_16

to bear the parents' fear,
to stand unshaken
in the long night
where their hope
rests entirely in him.

Building Trust in Pediatrics: A Journey of Care, Communication, and Connection

Pediatrics is more than a branch of medicine—it's a partnership in growth. It's where science meets storytelling, where a child's first steps are mirrored by a parent's first fears, and where care begins long before the stethoscope touches the chest. Pediatricians aren't just healers; they're observers, educators, cheerleaders, and confidants. From the newborn's first cry to the teenager's first independent decision, pediatrics is a field built on relationships and rooted in trust (Fig. 16.1).

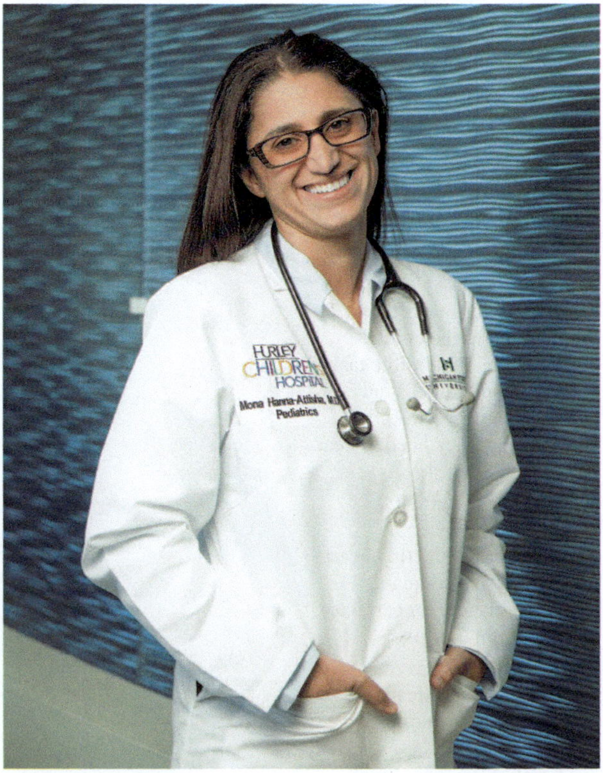

Fig. 16.1 Dr. Mona Hann-Attisha. (Photo courtesy of Mike Naddeo photography)She was awarded the Freedom of Expression Courage Award by PEN America and named one of Time magazine's 100 Most Influential People in the World for her role in uncovering the Flint Water Crisis. As a physician, she listened to her patients to understand their problems and recognize the cause of their illness

The Heartbeat of Pediatric Care: Trust

In pediatric care, trust isn't a luxury—it's a necessity. Unlike adults, children often can't articulate what's wrong. Instead, pediatricians must rely on a blend of intuition, creativity, and emotional intelligence to connect and diagnose. A toddler's appointment might include turning a stethoscope into a "magic listening tool" or making the otoscope a "treasure-hunting flashlight." These playful gestures are more than distractions—they're trust-building rituals that create a safe space for children. As children grow, their trust evolves too. School-aged kids begin to engage more directly, asking questions and participating in their own care. By the teenage years, the pediatrician becomes more than a doctor—they become an ally. When teens feel heard and respected, they're more likely to open up, take ownership of their health, and carry those habits into adulthood.

Navigating the Parent-Child-Pediatrician Triangle

Pediatric care is rarely a one-on-one interaction. It's a triad—pediatrician, parent, and child—each with their own needs and concerns. Early on, parents are the voice and advocate for their child, but as children grow, so should their role in the conversation. A skilled pediatrician knows how to shift the dynamic gradually, creating a dialogue where both parent and child feel seen and heard. This balancing act becomes even more delicate with preteens and teens. Parents may still make the decisions, but teens need space to speak for themselves. Giving them a voice in their own care fosters confidence and builds health literacy, both of which are critical as they approach adulthood.

Caring for Teens: Respect, Privacy, and Empowerment

Teenagers are often the most complex patients—not because of their symptoms, but because of the unspoken emotions behind them. They're navigating identity, independence, and sometimes silence. A pediatrician who can offer nonjudgmental, honest dialogue becomes a powerful figure in a teen's life. Creating safe, confidential spaces for teens—particularly in discussions about mental health, relationships, or substance use—sends a strong message: *You matter, and you're in control.* When teens feel that autonomy, they're far more likely to share openly and follow through on care. Follow-ups, even simple ones—"*How are you feeling since our last visit?*" or "*Did that new strategy help?*"—reinforce that their voice carries weight, and their concerns won't disappear the moment they leave the exam room.

Supporting Parents: Compassion in Every Conversation

Behind every worried child is often an even more anxious parent. Pediatricians are not only treating symptoms—they're often addressing fears, doubts, and guilt. A calm, compassionate explanation can transform a parent's panic into understanding. This means more than just listing treatment options—it means listening fully, validating concerns, and providing clear, jargon-free guidance. Sensitive topics, like vaccine hesitancy, require particular care. Rather than confrontation, pediatricians must lean into education and empathy. By grounding the conversation in evidence—and treating parents with respect, not judgment—trust can be strengthened, even in disagreement.

Delivering Difficult News: Honesty with Hope

One of the hardest moments in any pediatrician's career is delivering bad news. These moments demand not only clinical clarity but deep emotional presence. While it's tempting to soften the message, leading with connection and actionable steps often has the greatest impact. Framing the conversation around "*Here's what we know, and here's what we're going to do together*" can be far more supportive than simply saying, "*I'm sorry*." Parents don't just need facts—they need hope, a plan, and reassurance that they're not facing this alone. Even in moments of uncertainty or grief, a pediatrician's steady presence can be a beacon.

Communication as a Healing Tool

In pediatrics, communication isn't just a skill—it's a form of medicine. Every smile, every question encouraged, every clear explanation delivered with empathy becomes part of the healing process. Whether explaining a complex treatment or soothing a child's pre-vaccine jitters, how something is said can be just as important as what is said. For young children, non-verbal cues—tone of voice, facial expression, body language—matter deeply. For teens, it's about creating a safe space where questions aren't just allowed but welcomed. And for parents, clarity and compassion go hand in hand to build confidence in the care their child is receiving.

A Lifelong Partnership in Health

Pediatricians are more than physicians. They are guides, mentors, and steadfast companions in a family's health journey. Their influence extends beyond prescriptions and growth charts—it shapes the way children understand their bodies, voice their needs, and approach healthcare for the rest of their lives. In the tapestry of a child's development, the pediatrician is a constant thread—offering reassurance during fevers, cheering victories at milestones, and standing firm during challenges. By building trust, communicating with intention, and showing up with empathy, pediatricians don't just treat—they transform.

17 Recognizing and Responding to Burnout and Moral Injury

What Is Burnout?

Burnout is a term that has become almost synonymous with healthcare, but it's often misunderstood [1]. In the context of medicine, burnout refers to emotional exhaustion, depersonalization (a sense of disconnection from patients), and a feeling of reduced personal accomplishment. Paradoxically, the very qualities that make healthcare workers compassionate and committed—empathy, a strong work ethic, and a desire to improve—are the same traits that can make them more susceptible to burnout. Burnout can appear at any stage of a healthcare career. It affects medical students, residents, fellows, and even seasoned physicians, particularly those who are deep into practice or research. Research shows that burnout rates are alarmingly high, especially among young physicians and, more concerningly, among female physicians. A survey of U.S. healthcare residents found that 42% reported burnout, and women were found to have an increased risk of burnout, with odds ranging from 20% to 60% higher than their male counterparts [2] (Fig. 17.1).

The consequences of burnout are far-reaching. It not only negatively affects healthcare providers' mental and physical health but also compromises patient care. Burned-out doctors are more likely to make medical errors, have reduced productivity, and experience higher rates of depression, substance abuse, and even suicidal ideation.

B. Silverman, *The Power of Bedside Manners in Patient Care*,
https://doi.org/10.1007/978-3-032-10496-0_17

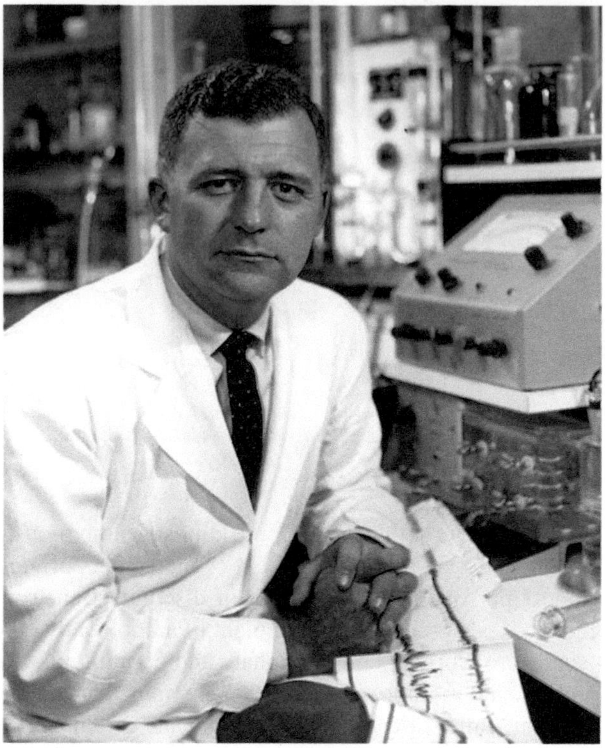

Fig. 17.1 Eugene Braunwald. (Photo courtesy of the Lillian and Clarence De La Chapelle medical Achieves at NYU)He grew up in Vienna and, in 1938 when Nazi Germany annexed Austria. His family fled and emigrated to New York City. 1972. He is an example of a life dedicated to medicine. Still active in his 90s he has been an outstanding clinician, scientist, and teacher. His life is a model of constantly remaking himself and continuing to contribute. It is an outstanding example for all healthcare workers

The Role of Moral Injury in Healthcare

Burnout in healthcare is intricately tied to a concept known as "moral injury," which arises when healthcare workers feel that they are unable to provide care in a way that aligns with their personal values [3, 4]. This feeling of moral conflict can stem from a variety of factors, including administrative burdens, the complexity of electronic medical records (EMRs), and the pressure of corporate healthcare environments that restrict physician autonomy.

Factors contributing to burnout:

1. **Asymmetrical Rewards**: Healthcare workers often receive little recognition for their hard work, while negative outcomes (especially bad patient outcomes) attract disproportionate blame and criticism.
2. **Loss of Autonomy**: Healthcare Providers face increasing micromanagement, restrictive time constraints, and pressure to adhere to standardized algorithms and excessive documentation. These factors erode their sense of professional control.
3. **Cognitive Scarcity**: Healthcare Providers are often forced to make difficult trade-offs when resources are limited, leading to decisions that may result in negative consequences. This strain is exacerbated by administrative demands that pull their attention away from patient care.

The process of delivering high-quality care has become more challenging. Medical treatments are increasingly complex, expectations for outcomes are higher, and administrative burdens (such as dealing with EMRs, insurance requirements, and other paperwork) take up more time than ever. Unfortunately, healthcare providers often lack organizational support systems to help them manage these challenges, leading to increased stress and a sense of helplessness.

How to Combat Burnout [5]

Individual Strategies

If you're feeling overwhelmed, it's critical to seek support. Find a mentor, a senior colleague, or a training director who can offer guidance and a listening ear. Sometimes, just changing your routine can provide a refreshing perspective. Try altering your schedule—changing the timing of when you see patients or when you perform certain tasks can reinvigorate your workday. Breaks are essential, too. Whether it's taking a coffee break, stepping outside for a walk, or even taking a longer break from work to reconnect with your family, stepping away from the grind can be crucial for emotional recovery. It's important to recognize the need to care for yourself. Helping others in a high-stress environment can be incredibly draining. Focusing on self-care and relaxation techniques—whether through exercise, meditation, hobbies, or simply taking time to rest—can go a long way toward preventing burnout.

Organizational Changes

Addressing burnout requires systemic change, not just individual effort. Organizations need to recognize the importance of creating a work culture that values well-being. This includes ensuring fair workload distribution, promoting transparent communication, and supporting flexible work schedules that respect work-home balance. Leadership should also create an environment where healthcare providers have the autonomy to make decisions and the opportunity for professional development.

Finding the Right Environment

When preparing for residency, fellowship, or your first post-training job, it's important to assess the organizational culture of the institutions you're considering. Key questions to ask include:

- Is the organization transparent with its communication, especially regarding expectations and resources?

- Does the institution foster collaboration, or is it more siloed and competitive?
- What are the opportunities for career advancement and personal development?
- Does the institution provide adequate support for work-life integration, such as parental leave and child care?
- Are wellness programs and burnout prevention strategies in place?

The right organizational culture can significantly reduce the risk of burnout and enhance overall job satisfaction.

Conclusion: Creating a Healthier Future for Healthcare Workers

The healthcare system is under tremendous strain, and burnout among healthcare workers is one of the most pressing issues facing the profession today. However, there is hope. By addressing both individual well-being and organizational culture, we can create a healthier, more sustainable healthcare environment. Whether through personal mindfulness practices, systemic organizational changes, or supportive leadership, the path forward requires a collective effort to ensure that healthcare professionals are not only able to provide the best care for their patients but also take care of themselves along the way.

References

1. West CP, Dyrbye LN, Shanafelt TD. Physician burnout: contributors, consequences and solutions. J Intern Med. 2018;283(6):516–29. https://doi.org/10.1111/joim.12752.
2. Kane L. Medscape national physician burnout & suicide report 2020: the generational divide. Available from: https://www.medscape.com. Accessed 16 Aug 2025.
3. Rabin S, Kika N, Lamb D, Murphy D, Stevelink SA, Williamson V, Wessely S, Greenberg N. Moral injuries in healthcare workers: what causes them and what to do about them? J Healthc Leadersh. 2023;15:153–60. https://doi.org/10.2147/JHL.S396659. PMID: 37605753; PMCID: PMC10440078.
4. Schnyder U. What is moral injury? Psychother Psychosom. 2024;93(6):367–71. https://doi.org/10.1159/000540679. Epub 2024 Aug 29. PMID: 39208779.
5. Maresca G, Corallo F, Catanese G, Formica C, Lo Buono V. Coping strategies of healthcare professionals with burnout syndrome: a systematic review. Medicina (Kaunas). 2022;58(2):327. https://doi.org/10.3390/medicina58020327. PMID: 35208650; PMCID: PMC8877512.

18 Bedside Manners: The Foundational Concepts, Values, and Assumptions Underlying the Practice of Medicine

Into whatever houses I enter, I will enter to help the sick, and I will abstain from all intentional wrongdoing and harm...

The Wisdom and Sagacity of Our Medical Forefathers

This chapter explores the timeless wisdom of physicians who profoundly shaped the doctor-patient relationship across history. Among the most influential are Hippocrates, John Gregory, Thomas Percival, William Osler, and Francis Weld Peabody. These pioneers understood that effective medicine extends beyond scientific knowledge—it also demands empathy, emotional intelligence, and clear communication. They championed the belief that physicians must not only diagnose and treat disease but connect with patients as fellow human beings.

This deeply relational approach—what we now call the *Art of Medicine*—acknowledges the emotional, psychological, and social dimensions of healing. It emphasizes that caring for patients is as much about listening and understanding as it is about tests and treatments (Fig. 18.1).

In today's high-tech healthcare environment—shaped by telemedicine, electronic records, and rapid innovation—it is more important than ever to remember that medicine remains a human endeavor. At its core lies the personal bond between doctor and patient. The enduring relevance of the Hippocratic Oath reflects this truth, calling on physicians to "do no harm" and to prioritize the well-being of those in their care. Its message of moral responsibility transcends centuries and continues to inspire ethical practice today [1].

This understanding of medicine as a human-centered vocation invites us to treat patients as whole persons, not just collections of symptoms. It challenges us to create spaces of trust and compassion where healing can begin—not just in the body, but in spirit and mind. By investing in the emotional well-being of those we serve,

B. Silverman, *The Power of Bedside Manners in Patient Care*,
https://doi.org/10.1007/978-3-032-10496-0_18

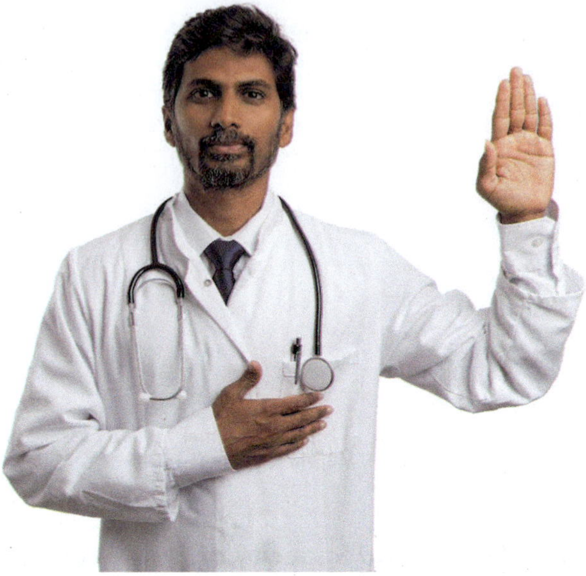

Fig. 18.1 Pledging the Hippocratic Oath

we improve not only patient satisfaction and treatment adherence, but overall health outcomes.

The wisdom of these early physicians serves as a guidepost in our modern world. No matter how far technology advances, the essence of healing remains rooted in compassion, respect, and integrity. As we navigate the complexities of contemporary medicine, we must stay grounded in these timeless principles, ensuring the doctor-patient relationship remains a sanctuary of empathy, trust, and human connection.

The Hippocratic Oath

I swear by Apollo the Healer, by Asclepius, by Hygieia, by Panacea, and by all the gods and goddesses, making them my witnesses, that I will fulfill according to my ability and judgment this oath and this covenant:

To hold him who has taught me this art as equal to my parents and to live my life in partnership with him, and if he is in need of money, to give him a share of mine, and to regard his offspring as equal to my brothers in male lineage and to teach them this art—if they desire to learn it—without fee and covenant;

To give a share of precepts and oral instruction and all the other learning to my sons and to the sons of him who has instructed me and to pupils who have signed the covenant and have taken an oath according to the medical law, but to no one else;

I will use those dietary regimens which will benefit my patients according to my greatest ability and judgment, and I will do no harm or injustice to them.

I will not give a lethal drug to anyone if I am asked, nor will I advise such a plan; and similarly I will not give a woman a pessary to cause an abortion.

In purity and according to divine law will I carry out my life and my art.

I will not use the knife, not even on sufferers from stone, but will withdraw in favor of such men as are engaged in this work.

Whatever houses I may visit, I will come for the benefit of the sick, remaining free of all intentional injustice,

The Hippocratic Legacy [2]

The **Hippocratic Oath**, attributed to the ancient Greek physician Hippocrates, is one of the oldest and most influential texts in the history of medicine. Though its language and specific prohibitions have evolved over time, its core values—ethical practice, patient welfare, humility, and professional responsibility—remain at the heart of modern medical ethics.

When first introduced around the fifth century BCE, the Oath was revolutionary. At a time when medicine was inconsistent and largely unregulated, it established a standard of conduct that elevated the practice from trade to moral vocation. By swearing allegiance to higher ideals and invoking divine witnesses, physicians pledged themselves to integrity and the service of others—not personal profit or prestige.

Patient-Centered Care

Central to the Oath is the principle of **primum non nocere**—"first, do no harm." This is more than a precaution; it is a mindset. It compels physicians to weigh their actions carefully, to avoid unnecessary interventions, and to protect patients from harm—whether physical, emotional, or psychological. The Oath also cautions against overstepping one's expertise, highlighting the importance of humility and collaboration in clinical care.

Professional Integrity and Lifelong Teaching

Equally important is the Oath's emphasis on **confidentiality, discretion, and mentorship**. Physicians are urged to uphold the trust patients place in them and to share knowledge only with those committed to the ethical practice of medicine. This call to teach responsibly reminds us that medicine is both a science and a tradition—passed from one generation to the next, not only through books and research, but through lived example and moral stewardship.

Relevance in the Modern Era

Though few physicians today recite the classical version of the Hippocratic Oath, its essence lives on in contemporary adaptations, such as the **Declaration of Geneva**. These modern iterations reaffirm the Oath's spirit in light of today's medical realities—from genetic engineering and end-of-life decisions to health disparities and digital privacy. The foundational principles of Hippocrates continue to offer clarity in moments of ethical uncertainty and moral complexity.

Medicine as a Moral Calling

The Hippocratic Oath remains more than a historical artifact—it is a living symbol of medicine's enduring commitment to humanity. It reminds us that, at its best, medicine is not just a profession, but a **calling**: one that demands compassion, courage, and a deep respect for the lives entrusted to our care. As we face new challenges in science, policy, and technology, the Oath challenges us to remain anchored in the values that first defined our calling—to heal, to serve, and above all, to do no harm (Fig. 18.2).

John Gregory: The Enlightenment and the Birth of Bedside Ethics

John Gregory, an eighteenth-century Scottish physician and moral philosopher, holds a unique place in the history of medicine. Living from 1724 to 1773, he helped lay the intellectual foundation for modern medical ethics and professionalism. Deeply influenced by the Scottish Enlightenment and thinkers like David Hume and Francis Hutcheson, Gregory brought a fresh moral seriousness to medicine at a time when the profession was still evolving its ethical identity.

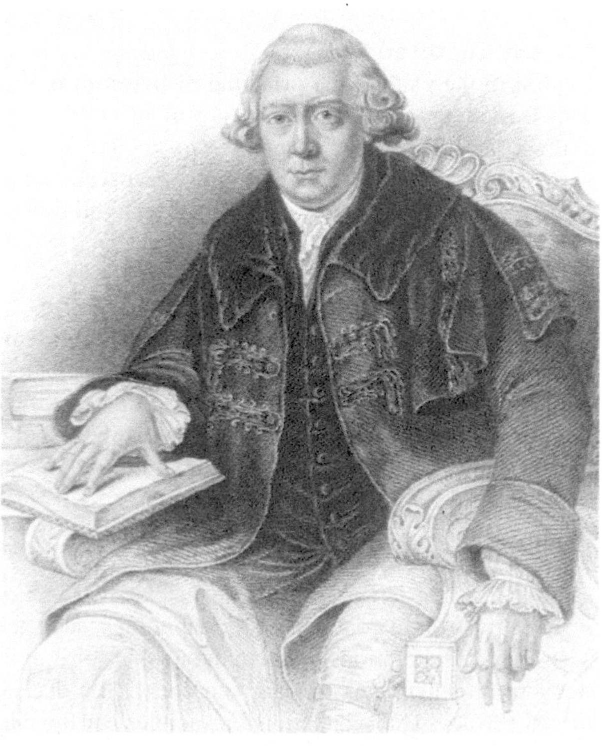

Fig. 18.2 John Gregory. ((from [x.y], licensed under CC-BY 4) Wellcome Trust Collection)

In 1770, Gregory delivered a series of lectures in Edinburgh titled *Observations on the Duties and Offices of a Physician, and on the Method of Prosecuting Inquiries in Philosophy* [3]. These were later transcribed by his students and published after his death. In them, Gregory sought not just to teach young doctors how to treat illness, but how to live as ethical physicians. He emphasized that medicine is not just a technical craft, but a moral calling—rooted in compassion, integrity, and public trust.

Gregory's ideas had a lasting influence. His work directly inspired Thomas Percival, whose 1803 book *Medical Ethics* became the model for the American Medical Association's first Code of Medical Ethics in 1847. Thanks to Gregory, medical ethics began to shift from unwritten tradition to a more formal and philosophical discipline—an approach that continues to shape medical education and bioethics today.

Gregory's Major Contributions to Medical Ethics

1. **Medicine as a Moral Practice**

   Gregory argued that medicine was more than diagnosing and curing disease. It required moral character—honesty, sympathy, and a genuine concern for the patient's well-being. Physicians, he believed, had a duty to serve both individuals and society with compassion and humility.

2. **Humanizing the Doctor-Patient Relationship**

   He challenged the view of patients as mere clinical cases. Instead, he promoted an empathetic approach, where physicians were expected to respect patients as persons—vulnerable, dignified, and deserving of care and understanding.

3. **Professional Conduct and Integrity**

   Gregory called for physicians to uphold high moral standards in both their public and private lives. He believed medicine should be seen not simply as a job, but as a vocation—a noble calling grounded in virtue and ethical responsibility.

4. **The Role of Sympathy (Empathy)**

   Gregory introduced the radical idea that emotional sensitivity was essential to good doctoring. Sympathy, or what we now call empathy, was not a weakness but a strength. This perspective marked a break from the cold, detached image of the physician and moved toward a more humane model of care.

5. **Foundations of Modern Medical Ethics**

   Many core principles Gregory introduced—confidentiality, beneficence, a duty to care for the poor—are still central to modern medical ethics. His ideas directly influenced later ethical codes and helped formalize the responsibilities expected of physicians.

Gregory and Today's Bioethics: A Comparison

1. **Autonomy**

   Modern View: Patients have the right to make informed decisions about their care. Autonomy, informed consent, and truth-telling are cornerstones of ethical practice.

   Gregory's View: He leaned toward **benevolent paternalism**. Gregory believed the physician, guided by moral insight, should act in the patient's best interest—sometimes even withholding distressing information to protect them.

   While modern ethics centers on patient choice, Gregory emphasized physician responsibility.

2. **Informed Consent**

   Modern View: Patients must be fully informed—about their diagnosis, risks, and alternatives—and freely consent to any treatment.

   Gregory's View: He supported honesty but advised discretion. Full disclosure, especially if it might upset the patient, was not always appropriate in his view.

   Today's emphasis on transparency contrasts with Gregory's protective stance, which prioritized emotional well-being over complete disclosure.

3. **Moral Character vs. Systemic Ethics**

   Modern View: Ethics now involves systems, structures, and laws—focusing on justice, accountability, and shared decision-making, not just personal virtue.

   Gregory's View: Ethics was a matter of personal integrity. The "good doctor" was someone who embodied moral values and treated medicine as a moral life.

   Gregory's focus on character still resonates, even as modern ethics has broadened to include social, legal, and institutional concerns.

Lasting Legacy

John Gregory was among the first to argue that physicians must not only be scientifically competent but also morally trustworthy. His *Observations on the Duties and Offices of a Physician* was a pioneering attempt to articulate a systematic code of ethics for doctors. He helped transform medicine from a trade into a profession—one grounded in trust, empathy, and moral duty. Though some of his views—especially his paternalism—differ from today's emphasis on patient autonomy, Gregory's central message endures: good medicine is as much about character and compassion as it is about knowledge and skill.

Excerpts from the wisdom of John Gregory;s Observations on the Duty and Offices of Physician and on the Method of Prosecuting Inquiries in Philosophy. I have included those comments that are as true today as in 1770 and represent the most meaningful observations on the impact of a physician's bedside manners.

The design of the office which I have the honor to hold in this university, is to explain the practice the physick; By which I understand, the art of preserving health, of prolonging life, and of curing disease. An art of great extent and importance; For which all your former studies were intended to qualify you; And indeed, it is only so far as they tend to qualify you for this, that are of consequence to you as physicians. On this occasion I think it needs to dwell on the utility and dignity of the medical art. Its utility was never seriously called in question; Every man who suffers pain or sickness will very gratefully acknowledge the usefulness of an art which gives him relief. People may dispute whether the physic, on the whole, does most good or mischief to mankind? Just as today with dispute whether the facility of reason confiding how it is often perverted really contributes to make human life more comfortable and happy? Whether a vigorous constitution and an early independent fortune are blessings or curse to those who possess them? Whether the art and science in general have proved beneficial or detrimental to mankind? Such questions afford opportunities for the display of elegance, and for saying plausible and ingenious things; but still nobody doubts the real influential advantage attending those acquisitions, if the natural and proper use are made of them.................... Accordingly, it has been pointed against them with so much keenness, that we never meet with the physician in a dramatic representation, but he is treated as a solemn coxcomb and a fool. But it is very evident, that all this fanfare is levelled against the particular manners of the individuals, and not against the profession of medicine itself. Of the dignity of the profession, I need say very little. To excel in it requires a greater compass of knowledge that is necessary in any other.

Art. A knowledge of the mathematics, at least of the elementary parts of them, of natural history, and of natural philosophy, are sufficiently conducted within it, as well as the sciences of anatomy, botany, and chemistry, which are deemed it intimate branches. There are likewise some forms of knowledge, which though absolutely necessary to the function of the practice of medicine, are of such ornamental acquisitions as no physician who has had regular education is found without; Such are an acquaintance with Latin, Greek, and the French languages. If you add to this, that knowledge of the world, of men, and of manners, so useful to a physician, and which he naturally and insensibly imbibed from an extensive intercourse with mankind, I think it will evidently appear, that no profession requires a greater variety of liberal accomplishments than that of the physick. And this sufficiently establishes the dignity of the science.............

Besides the general consideration of the utility and dignity of the science of medicine, it may be considered in two different views.

1. In the first place as presenting a very ample field for the exertion of genius. The great extent of the subject and the variety of causes, which I shall afterwards endeavor particularly to explain, have left it imperfect in many of its parts, and indeed there are some paths in it hitherto untold.

2. In the second place, medicine prefers an equally extensive field for the execution of humanity and has numerous opportunities of giving that relief to distress, which the wealth of India could not purchase. This, to a benevolent mind must be one of the greatest pleasures that can ever hope to enjoy. But besides the good which the physician has often in its power to do in consequence of the skill in his profession there are many occasions that call for his influence as a man, as a man who feels for the misfortunes of his fellow creatures. In this respect he has many opportunities of displaying patients, good nature, generosity, compassion, and all the gentler virtues that do honor t human nature. I do not hear speak of the obligations of principle. I speak only of what nature dictates to a heart possessed of a portion of goodness and fidelity.................... Habit may beget a command of temper, and a seeming composure which is often mistaken for insensibility. When the insensibility is real, it is a great loss to a physician, as it deprives him of one of the most natural and powerful incitements to extract himself for the relief of his patient. On the other hand, a physician of too delicate sensibility is often rendered incapable of doing his duty by anxiety and an excess of sympathy, which cloud his understanding, depresses his spirit, and prevents him from acting with the steadiness and vigor, upon which the life of his patient in a great measure depends..............

That medicine may be considered either as an art the most beneficial and important to mankind, or as a trade by which a considerable body of men gain their substance. These two views, though distinct, are far from being incompatible, though in fact they are too often made so. I shall endeavor, however, to set this matter in such a light as may show that the system of conduct of a physician, which tends most to the advancement of his art, is such as will most efficiently maintain the true dignity and honor of the profession, and will even promote the private interest of each of its members as are men of real capacity and merit.......

In the prosecution of this subject, I shall in the first place, consider, what kind of genius, understanding and temperament naturally fit a man for being a physician. In the second place what are the moral qualities to be expected from him and the execution of his profession, the obligations of humanity, patience, attention, discretion, secrecy, and honor, which he lies under to his patience. In the third place, I shall take notice of the decorum and attentions particularly incumbent on him as the physician, and which tend most sufficiently to support the dignity of the profession; As likewise the general propriety of his manners, his behavior to his patients, to his brethren, to surgeons and apprentices......

I begin with an inquiry into the genius, understanding, and temper, which naturally fit a man for being a physician. Perhaps no profession requires so comprehensive a mind as medicine.........

Among the infinite variety of facts and theories with which his memory has been loaded in the course of the liberal education, it is his business to make a judicial separation between those founded in nature and experience, and those which owe their birth to ignorance, fraud, or the capricious systems of a heated and diluted imagination................ It will be unfortunate however for its patience, if a little experience does not humble this pride, and satisfy him that in many cases he neither knows the approximate causes nor the indications of cure, nor how to fulfill those indications when he does know them; Or show him, what is equally perplexing, that indications are different and contradictory...............

But although a physician should possess that enlarged medical genius, which I have this now described, a capacity of another kind is also required. A physician has not only his own prejudice to conquer, but he must study the temper and the struggle of the prejudices of his patient, of the relations, of his own brethren, of the world in general; he must guard himself against all the offences of those, whose interest interfere with his; And it unfortunately happened, that the only judges of his medical merit are those who have an interest in concealing or depreciating it. Hence appears the necessity of physician having a large share of common sagacity, and knowledge of the world, as well as medical genius and erudition..................

I come now to mention those moral qualities particularly required in the character of a physician. The most obvious of these is humanity; The sensibility of the heart which makes us feel for the difficulties of our fellow creatures, and which of consequence incites us in the most powerful manner to relieve them. Sympathy produces an anxious attention to a thousand little circumstances that may tend to relieve the patient; an attention which money can never purchase. Hence the unspeakable advantages of having a friend for a physician. Sympathy naturally engages the affection and confidence of a patient, which in many cases is of the utmost importance to his recovery. Physician possesses softness and gentleness of manner, a compassionate heart, and what Shakespeare so emphatically calls "the milk of human kindness," a patient feels his approach like that of a guardian Angel ministering to his relief; While every visit to a physician who is unfeeling, hard or brutal in his manners, makes his heart sink within him, as at the presence of one, who is come to pronounce his sentence of death....... Real sympathy is never ostentatious, On the contrary, it always strives to conceal itself................ Universal experience demonstrates, that a gentle and humane temper, so far from being inconsistent with the vigor of mind, is usual attendant; And that rough, blustering manners very generally accompany a weak understanding and a dastardly foul, and are indeed frequently affected my men void of magnanimity........................

There is a species of good nature different from the sympathy I have been speaking of, which is amiable in a physician. It consists in a certain gentleness and flexibility, which makes him suffer with patience, and even apparent cheerfulness, the many contradictions and disappointments he is subject to in his practice. If he is extremely rigid in particular in his directions about regimen, he may be assured that they will not be strictly followed; And if he is severe in his manners, the deviations from his rules will certainly be concealed from him. The consequence is, that he is kept in ignorance the true facts of his patient; He ascribes to the consequences of the disease, what is merely owing to the irregularities in diet, and attributes effects to medicines which were every day thrown out the window. The dangerous errors which in this way he may be led into, are sufficiently obvious, and might easily be prevented by a prudent relaxation of the rules which will never be obeyed..............

A prudent physician should therefore prescribe such laws, as, though not be the best, are, yet the best that will be obeyed. Of the different evils he should choose the least and, at any rate, never lose the confidence of his patient and thus be deceived as to the true situation.................

There is a numerous class of patients who put the physician's good nature and patience to a very severe trial; These I mean are patients who suffer from nervous complaints. Although the fears of these patients are generally groundless, yet their sufferings are real; And the disease is as much seeded in the constitution as rheumatism or dropsy. To treat it with ridicule or neglect, from supporting it the effect of a crazy imagination, is equally cruel and absurd.

We sometimes see a very remarkable difference between the behavior of physician at his first setting out in life, and afterwards when he is fully established in reputation and practice. When beginning the world, he is affable, polite, humane, and assiduously attentive to his patients, but when in process of time he has reaped the fruits of such a behavior, and finds himself above the world, an independent, he assumes a very different tone, he becomes haughty, capricious, careless, and sometimes perfectly brutal in its manners………… A physician, by the nature of its profession, has many opportunities of knowing the private characters and the private transactions in families. Besides what he learns from his own observation, he is often admitted to the imminent confidence of those, who perhaps think they owe their life to his care. He sees people in the most disadvantageous circumstances very different from those in which the world views them, oppressed with pain, sickness, and low spirits. In these humbling situations, instead of the usual cheerfulness, evenness of temper, and vigor of mind, he meets with peevishness, impatience, and a spirit perfectly broken and eventuated. Hence it appears how much the characters of individuals and the peace and happiness of families may sometimes depend on the direction, secrecy, and honor of a physician, who without deviating from truth, may render characters that are truly respectable, ridiculous and contemptible. …………………. I may mention among the moral duties' incumbent on a physician, that candor, which makes him open to conviction, and ready to acknowledge and rectify his mistakes. His obstinate adherence to an unsuccessful method of treating a disease may sometimes be owing to a high degree of self-conceit, and an absolute belief in the infallibility of his system. The era here is without remedy, because it flows from a weak and ignorant head. Profound knowledge and clear discernment may lead one into the extreme of dissidence and humility, that are absolutely inconsistent with self conceit. But it too often happens, that this obstinacy proceeds from a deficit in the heart. A physician sometimes sees he is wrong, but is too proud, or rather too vain, to acknowledge the error, specifically if the error is pointed out to him by another. To this species of pride, a pride incompatible with true dignity and elevation of the mind, have the lives of thousands been sacrificed. A prudent regard indeed for the patient's safety may often make it necessary for a physician to conceal any embarrassment or mistakes from him, least it harm him and loss his confidence; But no man will profit in an error he is conscious of, who has least regard to honour or principle……………………..

Sometimes a patient himself or sometimes one of his friends, will propose to the physician a remedy, which, for some reason or another, they expect may do him service. Their proposal may be a good one; It may suggest to the ablest Physician, what, perhaps, till then, might not have occurred to him. It is undoubtedly, therefore his duty to adopt it. Yet there are some of our faculty who, from a pretended regard to the dignity of the profession, but in reality from the meanest and most selfish views, refused to apply any remedy proposed in this manner, without regard to its propriety. But this is an indolent piece of tyranny. Every man has a title to speak where his life or his health is concerned, and every man is entitled to suggest would he thinks may save the life of his friend........................ If he really approves it, he should frankly say so, and act; accordingly, If he disapproves it, he should declare his disapprobation in such a manner, as shows it proceeds from conviction, and not from pique or obstinacy. If a patient is determined to try an improper or dangerous remedy, a physician should refuse his sanction; but he has no title to complain of his advice not being followed, as he has no right to hinder any man from going out of the world in his own way........................

Let me here extort you against a barbarous custom of some physicians, believing your patients when their life is absolutely the spirit of, and when it is no longer decent to take fees. It is as much the business of the physician to alleviate pain, and to soothe the avenues of death, as to cure disease. Even in cases where his skill as a physician can be of no further avail, his presence and assurance as a man and as a friend may be highly grateful and useful, both to the patient and his nearest relations. Neither is there any propriety in his going out at one door when the clergyman enters at the other; a quaint conceit of some in our faculty, more expressive of impiety than honor. On the contrary, it is decent and proper that they should mutually understand and assist one another. The conversation of a clergyman of cheerful propriety and good sense, in whom a sick man confides, may sometimes be of more consequence in comforting the anguish of his mind, and his spirits, than all the drugs in the dispensary, while a gloomy and wrongheaded behavior may terrify him to distraction, and cut short a life which, by proper attention there was the greatest probability of saving....................

There are often unhappy jealousies and animosities among physicians, from which their patients suffer very severely. A physician, however, who has any sense of justice or humanity, will never involve his patient in the consequences of private quarrels, with which he has nothing to do............ Many advantages arise from physicians consulting together, who are men of candor, usually confident of each other's honor. A remedy may occur to one which did not occur to another; And the physician may want resolution, or sufficient confidence in his own opinion, to prescribe a powerful but dangerous remedy, on which, however, the life of his patient may depend, in this case the concurrent opinion of his brethren may determine his conduct. .... The quarrels of physicians, when they end in appeals to the public, generally hurt all the contending parties; but what is a much more consequence they discredit the profession, and expose the whole faculty to ridicule and contempt..................... It is a physician's duty to do everything in his power, that is not morally criminal, to save the life of his patient, and to search for remedies from every source, and from every hand, however mean, and in many respects contemptible. ....

Among the peculiarity quorums of physician's character, much regard has been had to a certain formality in dress, and a peculiar gravity and statement in the general course of his behavior. I formally observed, that decorum and propriety have their foundation sometimes in nature and common sense, sometimes only in Caprice and fashion..................

The case is very different in the profession of medicine. There is no natural propriety in a physician wearing one dress in preference to another; It not being necessary that any particular respect or authority should be annexed to his office, independent of what his personal merit commands. Experience, indeed, has clearly shown, that all our external formalities have often been used as snares to impede on the weakness and credibility of mankind; That they in general have been most prospectively adhered to by the most ignorant and imprudent of the profession; And that they frequently supplant real worth and genius; And that so far from supporting the dignity of the profession, they often expose it to ridicule and contempt. If then there is no natural and real propriety in a physician wearing a distinguishing dress, he can be under no obligation to use it, but what arises from the peculiar fashion of the country where he resides. .... There is great impropriety in the physician indulging himself in a certain nicety and refined delicacy, which makes him easily disgusted with the many disagreeable circumstances he must meet within his practice. Genuine delicacy is the virtue of the mind, and though it flows itself by an attachment to cleanliness, neatness, and even elegance, where it can be afforded, yet it always gives place and forgets itself, where duty or the interest of humanity require it. It is ridiculous in a physician to think any attentions, or any duties, below his dignity, which can contribute to the relief of his patient. When necessity requires it, he acts unworthily, if he does not become, to the best of his abilities, both surgeon, apothecary, and even nurse. ....

I shall now, with the same freedom, comment on a circumstance not infrequent in the behavior of learned men, physicians as well as others, which seems to me very efficiently injurious to the true dignity of our profession; I mean the severity of manners, that abject flattery of people of rank and fortune, which in modern times, so often disgraces men, in other aspects eminent for learning and ingenuity. This is one of the most humbling circumstances in the general character of men of genius and science. The external magnificence and splendor which surround high rank, seems to dazzle the understandings of those who live at a distance from it, and who are ignorant what a contemptible insight it often covers. It makes them crouch to those outward distinctions of title and fortune, which their philosophy if it has anything but a name, would make them despise, at the same time that they paid them that external respect, which the order of society and the established forms of good breeding required............ If such pride, however, is not attended with good insolence, but is properly corrected by good nature or good manners, it is a very pardonable weakness, as it arises from qualities that ought to confer real rank and importance upon those who possess them....................

Experience certainly shows that mankind are wonderfully attached to whatever has an air of mystery and concealment. A vendor of a quack medicine does not tell more lies about its extraordinary virtues, than numbers of people do who have no interest in the matter, even men of undoubted sense and propriety. A passion for what is new and marvelous, operates more or less on every human imagination, and in proportion as that is heated, the understanding is duped and confounded.

When a nostrum is once indulged and sold for a trifle, all its wonderful qualities immediately vanish, and in a few months it is utterly forgot. If it is really a valuable medicine, the regular faculty may adopt it, but it never recovers its high reputation in the world. It is likewise said that this is the only way in which valuable medicine can be efficiently introduced into practice; Because it is the only way by which it can procure the attention of the public, or fair trial of its virtue; that the bulk of mankind will much more readily follow the directions of a man who professes to cure them by mysterious means, then by a regular physician, of established honor and capacity, who prescribes such plain things as their own common sense show them the propriety of. It is further alleged, that some of the best remedies in medicine were originally introduced as secrets through discredited by the regular physicians. But allowing for this to be true, yet as I have persuaded, that these nostrums on the whole, do much more hurt than good to mankind; That they hinder the advents of the art, are making people neglect what is known and established, in pursuit of what is unknown and never to be indulged; That by heating the imagination, they impede on the judgment and confound the science with a multitude of false facts; And that, from there being generally kept in the hands of worthless and illiterate men, who prescribed them indiscriminately, they are one of the greatest public nuisances under which we labor in Great Britain……..

But there are some peculiar circumstances in the profession of a physician, which should naturally dispose him to look beyond the present scene of things and engage his heart on the side of religion. He has many opportunities of seeing people, once the gay and the happy, sink into deep retired distress; Sometimes devoted to a certain, but punishable and lingering death; Sometimes struggling with bodily anguish, or the still fiercer tortures of a distracted mind. Such affirmative senses, one should suppose might soften any heart, not dead to every feeling of humanity, and make it reference that religion which alone can supplement the soul in the most complicated difficulties, that religion which teaches to enjoy life with cheerfulness, and to resign it with dignity, a physician who has the misfortune to be cut off from the happy prospect of security, if he has a good nature, will conceal his sentiments from those under his charge, with as much care as he would preserve them from the inspection of a mortal disease. Fortified with insensibility, or ardent in the pursuits of business or pleasure, he may not feel in how forlorn and melancholy a situation he himself has placed; But it is barbarous to deprive expiring nature of its last support, and to blast the only surviving comfort of those who have taken a last farewell of every solitary pleasure in connection. If motives of humanity, and regard to the peace and happiness of society, cannot restrain a physician from expressing sentiments destructive of religion or morals, it is vain to plead the obligations of politeness and decency of his profession. The most favorable construction we can put on such conduct, is to support, that it proceeds from an uncontrollable levity of mind or an unbounded vanity, then forgets all the ties of morals, decency, and good manners…………… (Fig. 18.3)

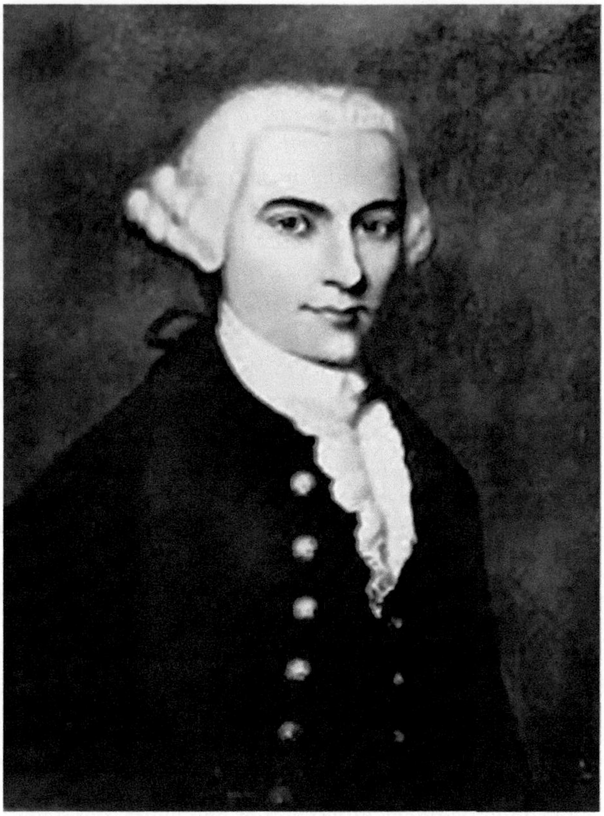

Fig. 18.3 Thomas Percival. ((from [x.y], licensed under CC-BY 4.0)" Wellcome Trust Collection)

Thomas Percival: A Pioneer in Medical Ethics and Medical Etiquette

Thomas Percival was an influential English physician and medical writer whose contribution significantly shaped the field of medical ethics. His seminal work, *medical ethics* [4], published in 1803, stands is one of the first comprehensive texts in systemically exploring the moral responsibility of physicians. In his groundbreaking book, Percival underscored the importance of professional conduct, patient care, and the physician's duty to society, setting a foundational framework for ethical medical practice.

Percival's writings focused on the principles of jurisprudence and medical etiquette, particularly emphasizing the nature of the physician patient relationship. His insights played a critical role in shaping the American Medical association's first code of medical ethics in 1847, making him a pivotal figure in the establishment of medical ethics within the medical profession. His legacy resonates through the development of subsequent medical codes of ethics that emerged throughout the 19th and 20th centuries, influencing how healthcare professionals engage with patients, colleagues, and the broader community.

The Evolution of Ethical Concepts from Percival's Times to Today

While Percival laid the groundwork for many modern ethical principles, the context and emphasis of medical ethics have evolved significantly since its time. Here are some of the key areas of development

1. **Professionalism and ethics**: Percival strongly advocated for professionalism and ethical conduct among physicians, focusing on their moral obligations to patients and society. Today, while those principles remain vital, contemporary medicine also embraces broader understanding of patient rights, informed consent, and shared decision making. Physicians now actively involve patients in their care, recognizing their autonomy in individual preferences
2. **Patient autonomy**: In Percival's era, medical practice was predominantly paternalistic, with physicians often making decisions on behalf of patients under the assumption that they knew what was best. In stark contrast, modern medicine prioritizes patient autonomy, empowering individuals to participate actively in decisions regarding their health. The principle of informed consent is now fundamental, ensuring that patients are fully informed about their options and can make choices that reflect their values and beliefs.
3. **Holistic care**: While Percival acknowledged the significance of a patient's overall well-being, his perspective was largely centered on the responsibilities of the physician. Contemporary medical practice, however, adopts a more holistic approach that addresses not only the physical aspects of health but also the emotional, psychological, and social dimensions. Modern health care emphasizes collaboration among various professionals to provide comprehensive care that considers all aspects of a patient's life.

The following are Percival's own words on the doctor patient relationship and bedside manners.

In the preface to medical ethics Percival comments; *it is characteristic of a wise man to act on determinate principles; and the good man to be assured that they are comfortable to rectitude and virtue. The relation in which the physician stands to its patients, to his brethren, and to the public, are complicated and multifarious; involving much knowledge of human nature, and extensive moral duties. The study of professional ethics, therefore, cannot fail to invigorate and enlarge your understanding, whilst the observance of the duties which they enjoy, will soften your manners, expand your affections, conform you to that propriety and dignity of conduct, which are essential to the character of a gentleman.*

Percival's comments concerning the patient's feelings and emotions. *The feelings and emotions of the patient, under critical circumstances, require to be known and to be attended to, no less than the symptoms of their diseases. Thus, extreme timidity, with respect to venous action, counter indicates its use, in certain cases and constitutions. Even the prejudices of the sick are not to be condemned or opposed with harshness. Were those silenced by authority, they will operate secretly and forcefully on the mind, creating fear, anxiety, and watchfulness. As misapprehension may magnify real evils, or create imaginary ones, no discussion concerning the nature of the case should be entered into before the patient, either with the house surgeon, the pupils of the hospital, or any medical visitor.*

In the large wards of an Infirmary the patient should be interrogated concerning their complaints, in a tone of voice which cannot be overheard. Secrecy, also, when required by peculiar circumstances, should be strictly observed. Females should always be treated with the most scrupulous delicacy to neglect or to not support their feelings is cruelty; And every wound thus inflicted tends to produce a callousness of mind, a contempt of decorum, and an insensibility to modesty and virtue. Let these considerations be forcefully and repeatedly urged on the hospital pupils.

The moral and religious influence of sickness is so favorable to the best interests of men in society, that it is justly regarded as an important object in the establishment of every hospital. The institutions for promoting it should, therefore be encouraged by physicians and surgeons, whenever seasonable opportunities occur. And by pointing out these to the officiating clergy, the sacred office will be performed with propriety, discrimination, and a greater certainty of success. The character physician is usually remote either from the superstition or enthusiasm; And the aid, which he is now extorted to give, will tend to their exclusion from the sick wards of the hospital where their effects have often been known not only to be painful, but even fatal.

It may be necessary that a hospital patient, on the bed of sickness and death, should be reminded, by some friendly monitor of the importance of a last will and testament to his wife, children, or relatives, who otherwise, might be deprived of his effects, of his expected prize money, or some kind of future residuary legacy.

A physician should not be forward to make gloomy prognostication; because they savor of empiricism, by magnifying the importance of his services in the treatment or cure of a disease. But he should not fail, on proper occasions, to give to the friends of the patient, timely notice of danger, when it really occurs, and even to the patient himself if absolutely necessary. For the physician should be the minister of hope and comfort to the sick: that by such cordials to the drooping spirit, he may soothe the bed of death; Revive expiring life; And counteract the depressing influence of those maladies which robbed the philosopher of fortitude, and the Christian of consolation.

References

1. Sioutis S, Reppas L, Bekos A, Limneos P, Saranteas T, Mavrogenis AF. The Hippocratic oath: analysis and contemporary meaning. Orthopedics. 2021;44(5):264–72. https://doi.org/10.3928/01477447-20210819-08. Epub 2021 Sept 1.
2. Sigerist HE. The great doctors. Hippocrates. New York: Dover Publications Inc.; 1971. p. 29–38.
3. Gregory J. Observations on the duties and offices of a physician; and on the method of prosecuting enquires in philosophy. ECCO print Editions Reprinted from the British Library London printed by W. Strahan and T. Cadell; 1770.
4. Perical T. Percival's medical ethics. Columbia: Leopold Classic Library; 2025.

19 The Gentle Art of Healing: Twentieth Century Concepts of Bedside Manners in the Osler-Peabody Tradition

Sir William Osler: Compassion, Equanimity, and the Heart of Medicine

Sir William Osler, often called the "father of modern medicine," helped shape the soul of modern medical practice—not just through scientific advancement, but by emphasizing compassion, empathy, and the humanity of caregiving. A pioneer of patient-centered care, Osler insisted that doctors look beyond symptoms to truly see the person suffering from the disease. His famous advice captures this ideal: *Care more particularly for the individual patient than for the special features of the disease* (Fig. 19.1).

Osler's influence on bedside care was transformative [1]. He believed that the best education for young physicians came not only from books, but from close observation of experienced clinicians—especially their demeanor. He taught that kindness, calmness, and humility were as important as clinical knowledge. For Osler, mentorship was not just the transmission of facts, but of values.

In his iconic 1889 address, "**Aequanimitas**," Osler urged physicians to develop emotional steadiness in the face of adversity—but never at the cost of compassion: *In men of the world, the calmer judgment and deeper sympathies are the fruit of age and experience... coolness and presence of mind under all circumstances, calmness amid storm, clearness of judgment in moments of grave peril... a divine gift.* He warned, however, that this calm—often mistaken for cold detachment—must be tempered by warmth: *Educate your nerve centers so that not the slightest dilator or contractor influence shall pass to the vessels of your face under any professional trial.* Osler's ideal physician balanced equanimity with empathy—not aloofness but composed compassion [2].

B. Silverman, *The Power of Bedside Manners in Patient Care*,
https://doi.org/10.1007/978-3-032-10496-0_19

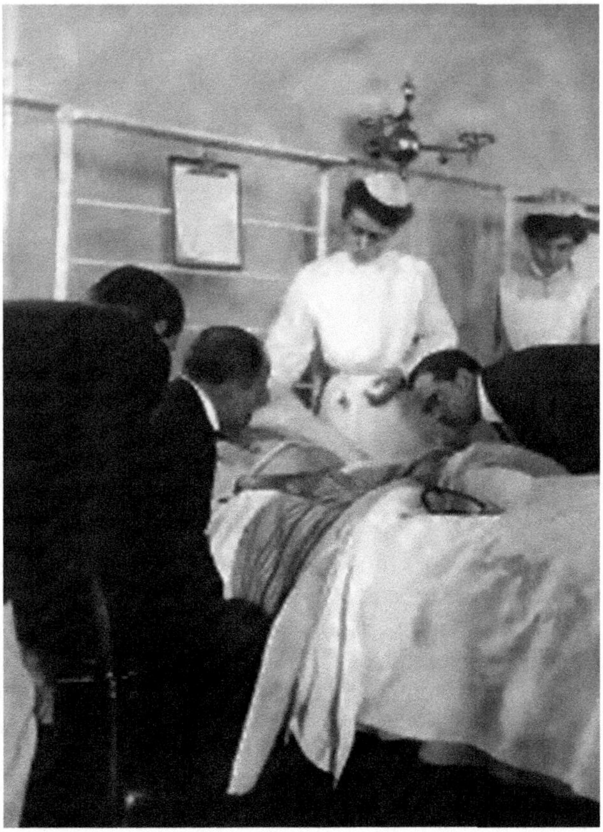

Fig. 19.1 William Osler at the Bedside. (Courtesy of the Mark Silverman Estate)

The Physician's Heart and Head

Osler placed great importance on cultivating not just the intellect but also the moral character of the physician: *Be careful when you get into practice to cultivate equally well your heart and your head.* He saw medicine as a calling, not a business—a sacred trust requiring emotional insight, ethical integrity, and selfless service: *The practice of medicine is an art, not a trade; a calling, not a business; a calling in which your heart will be exercised equally with your head. Our fellow creatures cannot be dealt with as men deal in corn and coal.* He acknowledged the unique demands of the profession: *The physician needs a clear head and a kind heart. His work is arduous and complex, requiring the exercise of the highest faculties of the mind while constantly appealing to the emotions and finer feelings.*

Treating the Patient, Not Just the Disease

Perhaps Osler's most enduring quote encapsulates his philosophy of medicine: *The good physician treats the disease; the great physician treats the patient who has the disease.* He urged doctors to listen deeply and observe carefully: *Listen to your patient, he is telling you the diagnosis.* He reminded students that every person is biologically and emotionally unique, and that true mastery involves a profound understanding of human nature: *Our study is man, as a subject of accidents or disease... To serve the art of medicine, as it should be served, one must love his fellow man.* He argued that science must be integrated with the old healing Art—never replaced by it: *It is much harder to acquire the art than the science... the old art cannot possibly be replaced but must be absorbed in the new science.*

Faith, Confidence, and the Healing Relationship

Osler also spoke eloquently of **faith**—not as dogma, but as a healing force rooted in trust: *As a profession—consciously or unconsciously, more often the latter—faith has been one of our most valuable assets.* He cited Galen, who noted that the physician who inspires the most confidence often heals most effectively. Especially in conditions we now call psychosomatic or functional, Osler believed the personal character of the physician could produce near-miraculous results: *Once let him gain the confidence of the patient, he can work with just the same sort of miracles as Our Lady of Lourdes. Nothing in life is more wonderful than faith... mysterious, indispensable, known only by its effect... faith pours out an unfailing stream of energy.* While he never claimed that faith could cure every illness, he saw it as a vital part of the healing relationship.

On the Afterlife and Humility

Though firmly grounded in science, Osler respected spiritual beliefs. He believed that even when unsupported by scientific proof, belief in a hereafter had real value: *In the presence of so many mysteries... he cannot be dogmatic and deny the possibility of a future state... a belief in the resurrection of the dead and a life of the world to come is the rock of safety to which many of the noblest of his fellows have clung.* Throughout his career, Osler remained humble, admitting *I've made mistakes, but they have been mistakes of the head, not of the heart.*

Osler's Legacy

Although Osler practiced in a very different era, his teachings remain profoundly relevant. He called for a kind, observant, and morally grounded practice of medicine, driven by both science and humanism. His legacy challenges today's clinicians

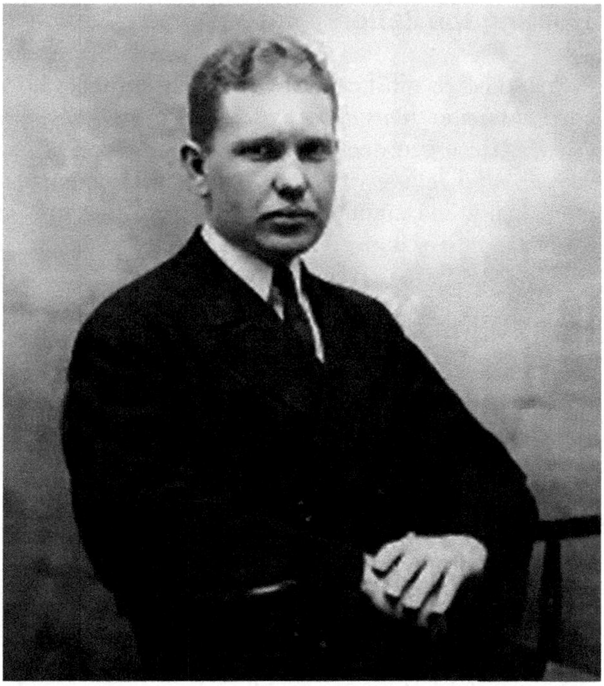

Fig. 19.2 *The Care of the Patient* by Frances Weld Peabody. (*JAMA March 19, 1927 used with copyright permission JAMA*. Courtesy of the Rockefeller Archive Center part of the Rockefeller University Records)

to remember that while medicine evolves, its essence remains unchanged: To treat not only the illness, but the person behind it—with skill, humility, and heart (Fig. 19.2).

In 1927, Francis Weld Peabody wrote a famous essay entitled "The Care of the Patient". which was delivered to the Harvard Medical student class [3]. It is worth considering what he said today as it remains as relevant to our care of patients today as it was then.

He comments: *our system of medical education is generally criticized and that the most common complaint is that our young graduates have been taught a great deal about the mechanisms of disease, but very little about the practice of medicine — or, to put it more bluntly, they are two "scientific" and do not know how to take care of patients. Many recent graduates encountered situations that they had not been led to anticipate and which they are not prepared to meet effectively. There is so much smoke, there is undoubtedly a good deal of fire, and the problem for teachers and for students is that to consider what they can do to extinguish what is left of the smoldering distrust. To begin with the fact must be accepted that one cannot expect to be a skillful practitioner of medicine in the four or five years allotted to the medical curriculum. Medicine is not a trade to be learned but a profession to be Entered. It is an ever-widening field that requires continued study and prolonged experience in close contact with the sick. All that a medical school can hope to do is to apply the foundations on which this is built. When one considers the amazing progress of science in the relationship to medicine during the past 30 years and the enormous mass of scientific material that must be made available to the modern physician, it is not surprising that schools have tended to concern themselves more and more with this phase of the educational problem. And while they have absorbed the difficult task of digesting and correlating new knowledge, it has been easy to overlook the fact that the application of the principles of science to the diagnosis and treatment of disease is only one limited aspect of modern practice. The practice of medicine in its broadest sense includes the whole relationship of the physician with the patient. It is an art, based to an increasing extent on the medical sciences, but comprising much of what still remains outside the realm of any science. The art of medicine and the science of medicine are not antagonistic but supplementary to each other. There is no more contradiction between science and medicine and the art of medicine then between the science of aeronautics and the art of flying. Good practice predisposes an understanding of the science which contribute to the structure of modern medicine, but it is obvious the sound professional training should include a much broader equipment. The problem that I wish to consider, therefore is whether the larger view the profession cannot be approached even under the conditions imposed by the current curriculum of the medical school. Can the practitioner's art be grafted on the main trunk of the foundational sciences in such a way that there may be symmetrical growth, like an expanding tree leaves which shall be for the healing of the nations. The physician speaks of the cure of patients is naturally thinking of circumstances as they exist in the practice of medicine; But the teacher who is attempting to train medical students is immediately confronted by the fact that even if he would, he cannot make the conditions under which he has to teach clinical medicine exactly similar to those of actual practice.*

The primary difficulty is the instruction has to be carried out largely on the wards and dispensaries of hospitals rather than in the patient's home and the physician's office. Now the essence of the practice of medicine it is an intensely personal matter and one of the chief difficulties between private practice and hospital practice is that the latter is always tends to be become impersonal. At the first sight this may not appear to be a very vital point, but it is, as a matter of fact, the crux of the whole situation. ***The treatment of the disease may be entirely impersonal; The care of the patient must be completely personal.*** *The significance an intimate personal relationship between the physician and patient cannot be too strongly emphasized, for in an extraordinarily large number of cases both the diagnosis and treatment are greatly dependent on it, and the failure of the young physician to establish the relationship accounts for much of this ineffectiveness in his care of patients.*

Hospitals like other institutions founded for the highest human ideals are not apt to deteriorate into dehumanized machines, and even the physician who has the patient's welfare most at heart finds the pressure of work forces him to give most of his attention to the critically ill and to those whose diseases are a menace to the public health. In such cases, he must first treat the specific disease and there remains little time in which to cultivate the more superficial personal contact with patients. Moreover, the circumstances under which the physician sees the patient are not wholly favored to the establishment of intimate personal relationship and this exists in private practice. One of the outstanding features of hospitalization is that it completely removes the patient from his customized environment. This may, of course, be entirely desirable, and one of the main reasons for sending a patient to the hospital to get him away from the home surroundings, which he is, be he rich or poor, are often unfavorable to recovery, but at the same time it is equally important for the physician to know the exact character of those surroundings.

Everybody, sick or well, is affected in one way or another, consciously or subconsciously, by the material and spiritual forces that bear on his life, and especially to the sick as forces may act as a powerful stimulants or depressants. When the General practitioner gets into the home of a patient he may know the whole background of the family life from the past experience, but even when he comes as a stranger, he has every opportunity to find out what manner of man this patient is, and what kind of circumstances make his life. He gets a hint of financial anxiety or domestic incompatibility; He may find himself confronted by the perilous, exacting, self-centered patient, or by a gentle invalid overawed by a dominating family; And as he appreciates how these circumstances are reacting on the patient, he dispenses sympathy, encouragement, or discipline. What is spoken of as a "clinical picture" is not just a photograph of a man and a sick in bed; It is an impressionistic pairing of the patient surrounded by his home, his work, his relatives, his friends, his joys, sorrows, hopes, and fears. Now, all of this background of sickness which bears so strongly on the symptomatology is liable to be lost sight of in the hospital: I say "liable to" because it is not by any means always lost sight of and because I believe that by making a constant and conscious effort one can almost always bring it out into its proper perspective. The difficulty is that in the hospital one gets into the habit of using the oil immersion lens instead of the lower power and focuses too intently on the center of the field.

When a patient enters the hospital, the first thing that commonly happens to him is that he loses his personal identity. He is generally referred to not as Henry Jones, but as "that case of mitral stenosis in the second bed on the left." There are plenty of reasons why this is so, and the point is, in itself, relatively unimportant; But the trouble is that it leads more or less directly to the patient being treated it's a case of mitral stenosis and not as a sick man. Disease is treated, but Henry Jones, lying awake nights while he worries about his wife and children, represents a problem that is much more complex than the pathophysiology of mitral stenosis, and is apt to improve very slowly unless a discerning intern discovers why it is that every large dose of digitalis failed to slow his heart rate. Henry happens to have heart disease, but he is not so disturbed as much by dyspnea as by anxiety for the future, and a talk with an understanding physician who tries to make the situation clear to him and then gets the social worker to find a suitable occupation, does more to straighten him out in a book full of drugs and diets. Henry has an excellent example of a certain type of heart disease; and he's glad that all of the staff find him interesting, for it makes him feel that they will do the best they can to cure him; Just because he is an interesting case, he does not cease to be a human being with very human hopes and fears. Sickness produces an abnormally sensitive morbid state in almost everyone, and in many cases the emotional state repercussions, as it were, on the organic disease. That pneumonia would probably run its course in a week, regardless of treatment, but the experience physician knows that by quieting the cough, getting the patient to sleep, and giving a bit of encouragement, he can save the patient his strength and lift him through many distressing hours. The institutional eye tends to become focused on the lung, and it forgets that the lung is only one member of the body.

But if teachers and students are inclined to take a limited point of view even toward interesting cases of organic disease, they fall much more serious error in their attitude toward a large group of patients who do not show objective, organic pathological conditions, and we're generally spoken of as having "nothing the matter with them." Up to a certain point, as long as they are regarded as diagnostic problems, they command attention; But as soon as the physician has assured himself, they do not have organic disease, he passes them over lightly.

Take the case of a young woman, for instance, who entered the hospital with a history of nausea and discomfort in the upper part of the abdomen after eating. Miss Brown had "suffered many things of many physicians." each of them gave her a tonic and limited her diet. She stopped eating everything that any of her physicians advised her to quit and is now living on a little milk with a few crackers; But her symptoms persist. History suggests a possible gastric ulcer or gallstones, and with a proper desire to study the case thoroughly, she is given a test meal, gastric analysis, duodenal intubation, and roentgen-ray examination are made of her gastrointestinal tract and gallbladder. All of these diagnostic studies give negative results; That is, they do not show incidence of any structural change. The case immediately becomes much less interesting than if it had turned out to be a gastric ulcer with atypical symptoms. The visiting physician walks by and says "well there's nothing a matter with her" the clinical clerk says "I did an awful lot of work on that case and it turned out to be nothing at all." the intern, wants to clear out the ward so as to make room for some interesting cases, says; "Missus b\Brown, you can send for your clothes and go home tomorrow. There is really nothing a matter with you and fortunately you have not got any of the serious problems we suspected. We have used all the most modern and scientific methods, and we find that there there's no reason why you should not eat anything you want to. I gave you a tonic to take when you go home." same story some colored medicine! Mrs. Brown goes home somewhat better for her rest in new surroundings, thinking that nurses are kind and physicians are pleasant, but they do not seem to know much about the sort of medicine that will touch her trouble. She takes up her life and the symptoms return and then she tries chiropractic, or perhaps Christian science.

It is rather fashionable to say that the modern physician has become "too scientific." Now, was it too scientific with all the stomach tubes and blood counts and X-ray examinations? Not at all. Miss Brown's symptoms might have been due to a gastric ulcer or gallstones, and after such a long course it was only proper to use every method that might help to clear the diagnosis. Was it, perhaps not scientific? The popular conception of a scientist as a man who works in a laboratory and who uses instruments of precision is inaccurate as it is superficial, for a scientist is known, not by his technical process, but by his intellectual process; and the essence of the scientific method of thought is that it proceeds in an orderly manner towards the establishment of a truth. Now the chief criticism to be made of the way Mrs. Brown's case was handled is that the staff was contented with a half-truth. The investigation of the patient was decidedly unscientific, and it stopped short of even an attempt to determine the real cause of the symptoms. As soon as organic disease could be excluded, the whole problem was given up, but the symptoms persisted. Speaking candidly, the case with a medical failure in spite of the fact that the patient went home with the assurance that there was "nothing the matter" with her. A good many "Miss Browns" male and female come to hospitals and a great many more go to private physicians. They're all characterized by the presence of symptoms that cannot be accounted for by organic disease and they are all liable to be told that they have "nothing the matter" with them. Now my own experience as a hospital physician and it's been rather long and varied and I've always found that from my point of view, hospitals are particularly interesting and cheerful places; but I'm fairly certain that except for a few low grade morons and some poor wretches who want to get in out of the cold, they are not many people who become hospital patients unless there is something the matter with them. And, by the same token, I doubt whether there are many people, except those stupid creatures who would rather go to the physician and go to the theater, we spend their money on visiting private physicians unless there is something the matter with them. In hospital and in private practice, however one finds the same type of patient and many physicians whom I have questioned agree in saying that excluding cases of acute infection, approximately half of their patients complained of symptoms for which an adequate organic cause could not be discovered. Numerically, then these patients constitute a large group, and their fees go a long way toward spreading butter on the doctor's bread. ***Medically speaking, they are not serious cases as regards perspective death, but they are often extremely serious as regards prospective life.*** *The symptoms will rarely prove fatal, but their lives will be long and miserable, and they may end by nearly exhausting their families and their friends. This is not the worst thing in the world, and to help a man to a happy and useful career maybe more of a service than saving a life.*

What is the matter with all these patients? Technically most of them come under the broad heading of the "psychosomatics"; But for practical purposes many of them may be regarded as patients with subjective symptoms due to disturbances of psychological activity of one or more of the organs or systems. These symptoms may depend on an increase or a decrease of a normal function, or an abnormality of a function or merely on the subjects becoming conscious of a woefully normal function that normally goes on unnoticed; And this last condition indicates that there is a close relationship between the appearance of these symptoms and the threshold of the patients' nervous reactions. The ultimate cause of these disturbances are to be found, not in the many structural changes of the organs involved, but rather in the nervous influences emanating from their emotional or the intellectual life, which, directly or indirectly effect in one way or another organs that are under either voluntary or involuntary control.

All of you have had experiences that have brought home the way in which emotional reactions affect ongoing functions. Some of you have been nauseated anxiously waiting for an important examination to begin, and even vomited; Others have been seized by an attack of diarrhea under the same circumstances. Some of you have had polyuria before making a speech, and others have felt an irregular pulse or a pounding tachycardia before a football game. Some of you have noticed rapid shallow breathing when listening to a piece of bad news, and others have known a type of occipital headache, with pain down the muscles of the back of the neck. It comes from nervous anxiety and fatigue. These are all simple examples of the way that emotional reactions may upset the normal functioning of an organ. Vomiting and diarrhea are due to abnormalities of the motor function of the gastrointestinal tract and to the production of an active revised peristalsis of the stomach and the relaxation of the cardiac sphincter, the other to hyper peristalsis of the large intestine. The polyuria is caused by vasomotor changes in the renal circulation, similar in character to the vasomotor changes that take place in the peripheral vessels and blushing and blanching of the skin, and in addition there are quite possibly associated changes in the rate of blood flow and in the blood pressure. Tachycardia and extra systoles, not only the rate but also the rhythm of the heart is under a nervous control that can be demonstrated in the intact human beings as well as in the experimental animal. The ventilatory function of the respiration is extraordinarily subject to nervous influences; So much so, in fact, that a study of the respiration in man is associated with peculiar difficulties. Rate, depth, and rhythm of breathing are easily upset by even minor stimuli, in extreme cases the disturbance in total ventilation is sometimes so great that gas is exchange becomes affected. Thus, I remember an emotional young woman who developed a respiratory neurosis with a deep and rapid breathing and expired so much carbon dioxide that the symptoms of tetany ensued. The explanation of the occipital headaches and so many pains in the muscles of the back is not entirely clear, but they appear to be associated with changes in muscular tone or with prolonged states of contraction. There is certainly a very intimate correlation between the mental tenseness and the muscular tenseness, and whatever methods are used to produce mental relaxation will usually cause muscular relaxation, together with relief of this type of pain. Similar condition is found in so-called writer's cramp, in which the painful muscles of the hand result, not from manual work, but from mental work.

One might go much further, but these few illustrations will suffice to recall the infinite number of ways in which the psychological functions may be upset by emotional stimuli, and the manner in which the resulting disturbances of function manifest themselves as symptoms. These symptoms, although obviously not due to anatomic changes, may, nevertheless be very disturbing and distressing, and there is nothing imaginary about them. Emotional vomiting is just as real as vomiting do the pyloric obstruction, and the so-called "nervous headaches" may be as painful as if they were due to a brain tumor. Moreover, it must be remembered that the symptoms based on functional disturbances may be present in a patient who has at the same time, organic disease and in such cases the determination of these causes is of different symptoms may be extremely difficult matter. Everyone accepts the relationship between common functional symptoms and nervous headaches, for convincing evidence is to be found in the fact that under ordinary circumstances the symptoms disappear just as soon as the emotional cause has passed. But what happened if the cause does not pass away? What if, instead of having to face a single three hour examination, one has to face a life of being constantly on the rack? The emotional stimulus persists, and continues to produce the disturbance of function. As with all nervous reactions, the longer the process goes on or the more frequently it goes on, the easier it is for it to go on. The unusual nervous track becomes an established path. After a time, the symptom and the subtle disorder that it produces comes to occupy the center of the picture, and the causative factors recede into a hazy background. The patient no longer thinks, "I cannot stand this life" but says out loud "I cannot stand nausea and vomiting. I must go to see a stomach specialist." quite possibly your comment on this will be that the symptoms of such neurotic patients are well known, and they ought to go to a neurologist or a psychiatrist and not to an internist or a general practitioner. In an era of internal medicine, however, which takes pride in the fact that it concerns itself with the functional capacity of organs rather than with mere structural changes, and which has developed so many "functional tests" of kidneys, heart, and liver, is it rather narrow minded to limit one's interests to disturbance of function which are based on anatomic abnormalities? There are other reasons, too why most of these "functional" cases belong to the field of general medicine. In the first place, the differential diagnosis between organic disease and pure functional disturbance is often entirely difficult, and it needs the broad training in the use of general clinical and laboratory methods which forms the equipment of the internist. Diagnosis is the first step in treatment. In the second place, the patients themselves frequently prefer to go to a medical practitioner rather than to a psychiatrist, and in the long run it is probably better for them to get straightened out without having what they often consider the stigma of having been "nervous cases." A limited number, it is true are so refractory or so complex that the aid of the psychiatrists must be sought, but the majority can be helped by the internist without highly specialized physiologic technique, if he will appreciate the significance of functional disturbances and interests himself in their treatment. The physician who does take these cases seriously one might say –scientifically- has the great satisfaction of seeing some of his patients get well, not as a result of drugs or as a result of the disease having run its course, but as a result of his own individual efforts.

Here, then, is a great group of patients which it is not the disease but the man or the woman who needs to be treated. In General Hospital practice physicians are so busy with the critically sick, and in clinical teaching they are so concerned with training students in physical diagnosis and attempting to show them all types of organic disease, that they do not pay much attention as they should to the functional disorders. Many a student enters upon his career having hardly heard of them except in his course in psychiatry, and without the faintest conception of how large a part they will play in its future practice. At best, his method of treatment is apt to be cheerful reassurance combined with the placebo. The successful diagnosis and treatment of these patients, however, depends almost wholly on the establishment of that intimate personal contact between physician and the patient which forms the basis of private practice. Without this, it is quite impossible for the physician to get an idea of the problems and troubles that lie behind so many functional disorders. If students are to obtain any insight into this field of medicine, they must also be given opportunities to build up the same type of personal relationship with their patients.

Is there, then, anything inherent in the conditions of clinical teaching and a General Hospital that makes this impossible? Can you form a personal relationship in an impersonal institution? Can you accept the fact that your patient is entirely removed from his natural environment and then reconstruct the background of the environment from the history, from the family, from a visit to the home or workshop, and from the information obtained by the social worker? And while you are building up this environmental background, can you enter into the same personal relationship that you ought to have in private practice? And if you can do all this, and I know from experience that you can, then the study of medicine in the hospital actually becomes the practice of medicine, and the treatment of disease immediately takes its proper place in the larger problem of the care of the patient.

When a patient goes to a physician usually has confidence that the physician is the best, or at least the best available, person to help him in what is, for the time being, his most important trouble. He relies on him as on a symptomatic adviser and a wise professional counselor. When a patient goes to a hospital he has confidence in the reputation of the institution, but it is hardly necessary to add that he also hopes to come into contact with some individual who personifies the institution and will also take a human interest in him. It is obvious that the first physician the patient sees is in the strategic position and in hospitals all students can have the satisfaction of being regarded as physicians.

Here, for instance, is a poor fellow who has just been jolted to the hospital in an ambulance. A string of questions about himself and his family has been fired at him, his valuables and even his clothes have been taken away from him, and he's wheeled into the ward on a truck, miserable, scared, defenseless, and in his nakedness unable to run away. He is lifted onto a bed becomes conscious of the fact that he is the center of interest in the ward, wishes that he had stayed at home among friends, and just as he is beginning to take stock of his surroundings, finds that the thermometer is being stuck under his tongue. It is all strange and new, and he wonders what is going to happen next. The next thing that does happen is that a man in a long white coat sits down beside by his bedside and starts to talk to him. Now, it happened that according to our system of clinical instruction that man is usually a medical student. Do you see what an opportunity you have? The foundation of your whole relationship with the patient is laid in these first few minutes of contact, just as happens in private practice. Here is a worried, lonely, suffering man and you begin by approaching him with sympathy, tact, and consideration, you get his confidence, and he becomes your patient. Interns and visiting physicians may come and go, and the hierarchy gives them a precedence; But if you make the most of your opportunities, he will regard you as his personal physician, and all the rest as mere consultants. Of course, you must not drop him after you have taken that history and made your physical examination. Once your relationship with him has been established, you must foster it by every means. Watch his condition closely and he will see that you are alert professionally. Make time to have little talks with him and these talks need not always be about his symptoms. Remember that you want to know him as a man, and this means you must know about his family, and his friends, his work and his play. What kind of person is he cheerful, depressed, introspective, careless, conscientious, mentally keen or dull. Lookout for all the little incidental things that you can do for his comfort. These two are part of "the care of the patient" some of them will fall technically into the field of nursing but you will always be profoundly grateful for any nursing technique that you have acquired. It is worth your while to get the nurse to teach you the right way to feed a patient, change the bed, or give a bed pan. Do you know the practical tricks that make a dyspneic patient comfortable? Assume some responsibility for these appropriately minor points and you will find it is when you are doing some such friendly service, rather than when you were being a formal questioner, that the patient suddenly starts to unburden himself, and a flood of light is then thrown on his situation.

Meanwhile, of course you will have been active along strictly medical lines, and by the time your clinical and laboratory examinations are completed you will be surprised to see how intimately you know him and everything you have picked up about him will be of value in the subsequent handling of the situation. Suppose, for instance, you find conclusive evidence that his symptoms are due to organic disease; Say a gastric ulcer. As soon as you face the problem of having out his regimen you find that it is one thing to write an examination paper on the treatment of gastric ulcer and quite another thing to treat John Smith, who happens to have a gastric ulcer. You want to begin by giving him rest in bed and a special diet for eight weeks. Rest means both nervous and physical rest. Can he get it best at home or in the hospital? What are the conditions at home? If you keep him in the hospital, it is probably good for him to see certain people, and bad for him to see others. He has business problems that must be considered. What kind of compromise can you make on them? How about the financial implications of eight weeks in bed followed by a period of convalescence? Is it, on the whole, wiser to try a strict regimen for a shorter period, and, if it does not improve, take up the question of operation sooner than is generally advisable? These and many similar problems arise in the course of treatment of most every patient, and they have to be looked at, not from the abstract point of view of the treatment of the disease, but from the concrete point of view of the care of the individual.

Suppose on the other hand that all your clinical and laboratory examination turn out entirely negative as far as revealing of any evidence of organic disease is concerned. Then you are in a difficult position of not having discovered the explanation of the patient's symptoms. You have merely assured yourself that certain conditions are not present, The first thing you have to consider is whether the symptoms are the result of organic disease in such an early stage that you cannot definitely recognize it. This problem is often extremely perplexing, requiring great clinical experience for its solution, and often you will be forced to fall back on time in which to watch developments. If, however, you finally exclude recognizable organic disease, and the probability of early or very slight organic disease, it becomes necessary to consider whether the symptomatology may be due to functional disorder which is caused by nervous or emotional influences. You know a good deal about the personal life of your patient by this time, but perhaps there is nothing that stands out at as an obvious ideologic factor, and becomes necessary to sit down for a long, intimate talk with him to discover what remains hidden.

Sometimes it is well to explain to the patient, by obvious examples, how it is that emotional states may may bring about symptoms similar to his own, so that he will understand what you are driving at and will cooperate with you. Often the best way is to go back to the very beginning and try to find out the circumstances of the patient's life at the time the symptoms first began. The association between symptoms and cause may have been simpler and more direct at the onset, at least in the patient's mind, for as time goes on, and the symptoms become more pronounced and distressing, there is a natural tendency for the symptoms to occupy so much of the foreground of the picture that the background is completely obliterated. Sorrow, disappointment, anxiety, self distrust, thwarted ideals or ambitions in social, business, or personal life, and particularly what are called the maladaptations to these conditions these are among the commonest and simplest factors that initiate and perpetuate the functional disturbances. Perhaps you will find that the digestive disturbances began at the time the patient was in serious financial difficulties, and that they have reoccurred whenever he is worried about money matters. Or you may find that 10 years ago a physician told the patient he had heart disease cautioning him "not to worry about it." For 10 years, the patient has never mentioned the subject, but he has avoided every exertion, and he's lived with the idea that sudden death was in store for him. You will find that physicians, by wrong diagnosis and ill-considered statements, are responsible for many a wrecked life, and you will discover that it is much easier to make a wrong diagnosis than it is to unmake it. Or, again, you may find that the pain in the woman's back made its appearance when she first felt her domestic unhappiness, and that this man's headaches have been associated, not with long hours of work, but with a constant depression due to unfulfilled ambitions. The causes are manifold and the manifestations protein. Sometimes the mechanism of cause and the effect is obvious; Sometimes it becomes apparent only after a very tangled scheme has been unrevealed.

If the establishment of an intimate personal relationship is necessary in the diagnosis of functional disturbances, it becomes doubly necessary in their treatment. ***Unless there is complete confidence in the sympathetic understanding of the physician as well as in his professional skill, very little can be accomplished****; but granted that you have been able to get close enough to the patient to discover the cause of the trouble, you will find that a General Hospital is not at all impossible place for the treatment of functional disturbances. The hospital has indeed, the advantage that the entire reputation of the institution and all that it represents in the very facilities for diagnosis and treatment, go to enhance the confidence which the patient has in the individual physician who represents it. This gives the very young physician a hold on his patients that they could scarcely hope to have without its support. Another advantage is that the hospital patients are removed from their* *usual environment, for the treatment of functional disturbances it's often easier when the patients are away from friends, relatives, home, work, and indeed, everything that is associated with their daily life. It is true that in a public ward one cannot obtain complete isolation in the sense that this is a part of the Weir Mitchell treatment, but the main object is accomplished if one has obtained the psychological effect of isolation which comes with an entirely new and unaccustomed atmosphere. The conditions, therefore, under which you, as students, come into contact with patients with functional disturbances are not wholly unfavorable, and with very little effort they can be made to simulate closely the conditions in private practice.*

It is not my purpose, however, to go into a discussion of the methods of treatment functional disturbances, and I have dwelt on the subject only because these cases illustrate so clearly the vital importance of the personal relationship between the physician and the patient and the practice of medicine. In all your patients whose symptoms are of functional origin, the whole problem of diagnosis and treatment depends on your insight into the patient's character and personal life, and in every case of organic disease there are complex interactions between the pathologic process and the intellectual process which you must appreciate and consider if you would be a wise clinician. There are moments, of course, in the case of serious illness when you will think solely of the disease and its treatment, but when the corner is turned and the immediate crisis is passed, you must give your attention to the patient. Disease in man is never actually the same as disease in an experimental animal, for in man the disease at once affects and is affected by all that we call the emotional life. Thus, the physician who attempts to take care of a patient while he neglects this factor is as unscientific as the investigator who neglects to control for all the conditions that may affect his experiment. The good physician knows his patients through and through, and his knowledge is brought dearly. Time, sympathy, and understanding must be lavished dispensed, but the reward is to be found in that the personal bond which forms the greatest satisfaction of the practice of medicine. ***One of the essential qualities of the clinician is interest in humanity, for the secret of the care of the patient is caring for the patient.***

The Evolution and Growth of Bedside Manners

This understanding of human nature and the importance of a meaningful doctor-patient relationship invites us to foster approaches that recognize patients as whole beings, not merely a set of symptoms. It challenges us to cultivate environments in which trust can flourish. By investing in the emotional well-being of patients, healthcare providers can not only enhance adherence to treatment but also improve overall health outcomes.

Ultimately, the wisdom of past physicians serves as a guidepost, reminding us that regardless of the advancements in medicine, the heart of healthcare remains a deeply human endeavor. Embracing this truth calls upon us to recognize our shared humanity and to practice medicine with compassion, integrity, and respect for the individual stories that every patient brings. As we continue to navigate the complexities of health care in contemporary society, we must remain grounded in these timeless principles, ensuring that the doctor-patient relationship remains a sanctuary of understanding and support amid the continual evolution of our field.

References

1. Silverman BD. Physician behavior and bedside manners: the influence of William Osler and the Johns Hopkins School of Medicine. Proc (Bayl Univ Med Cent). 2012;25(1):58–61.
2. Bryan CS. "Aequanimitas" Redux: William Osler on detached concern versus humanistic empathy. Perspect Biol Med. 2006;49(3):384–92. https://doi.org/10.1353/pbm.2006.0038. PMID: 16960308.
3. Peabody FW. The Care of the Patient. JAMA. 1927;88(12):877–82. https://doi.org/10.1001/jama.1927.02680380001001. Published Online: March 19, 1927.

20 The Nuremberg Code and the Belmont Report: The Guiding Principles of Human Research Ethics

The **Nuremberg Code** and **Belmont Report** represent the moral compass guiding modern medicine. They transformed medicine from paternalism to **patient autonomy, safety, and social justice**—fundamental values for every doctor today. They are both foundational documents in the field of medical ethics that have significantly shaped the conduct of research involving human subjects and established important principles for medical care and experimentation. As a healthcare provider it is important that you understand what these codes say and how important they are in our current practice of medicine (Fig. 20.1).

B. Silverman, *The Power of Bedside Manners in Patient Care*,
https://doi.org/10.1007/978-3-032-10496-0_20

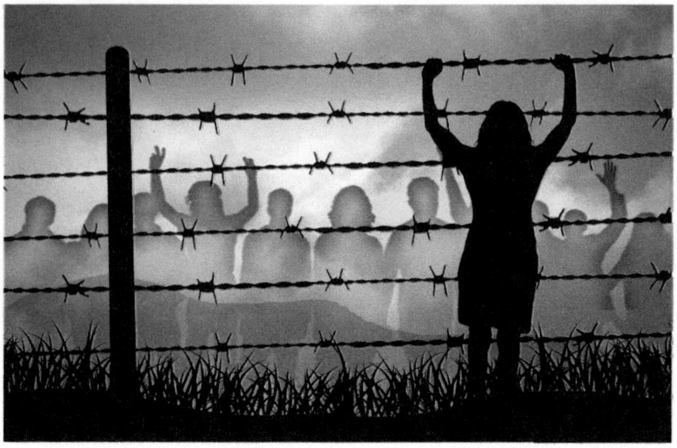

Fig. 20.1 Prisons of war

The Nuremberg Code [1]

Response to Historical Atrocities

The **Nuremberg Code** was born out of the horrific medical atrocities committed during **World War II**, particularly by Nazi physicians during the **Holocaust**. In concentration camps, doctors carried out brutal experiments on prisoners **without consent**, subjecting them to:

- Extreme temperatures
- Infectious disease exposure
- Forced sterilizations and eugenics procedures
- High-altitude and pressure testing

These were not medical trials—they were crimes against humanity.

In response, the **Nuremberg Trials** were held after the war to bring Nazi leaders to justice. One of these was **the Doctors' Trial,** where **23 Nazi doctors and administrators** were prosecuted by an American military tribunal in **Nuremberg, Germany,** between **December 9, 1946, and August 20, 1947**. The charges included **war crimes** and **crimes against humanity**, with a focus on the inhumane experiments conducted on innocent human subjects.

During the trial, American medical experts—most notably **Dr. Leo Alexander** and **Dr. Andrew Ivy**—played a key role in developing a new set of ethical guidelines. These became known as the **Nuremberg Code**, issued in **1947** as part of the court's final judgment.

The purpose of the Code was clear: to ensure that **no medical experiment would ever again be conducted without the voluntary and informed consent of the subject.** It established 10 foundational principles that have since shaped modern medical and research ethics around the world.

One of the key principles of the Nuremberg code is a necessity of voluntary and informed consent from all participants. This principle fundamentally shifted the approach to medical research ensuring that individuals have a right to make informed choices about their participation in studies.

Ethical Standards
The code outlines 10 essential principles for conducting research, including the necessity of scientifically valid research that should yield fruitful results for the good of society.

The 10 Essential Principles of the Nuremberg Code

1. **Voluntary Consent Is Essential**
   The voluntary, informed consent of the human subject is absolutely essential. Participants must have legal capacity, be able to exercise free choice, and understand the nature, purpose, and risks of the experiment.
2. **The Experiment Should Yield Beneficial Results**
   The experiment should aim to produce results for the good of society that cannot be obtained by other methods.
3. **It Must Be Based on Prior Knowledge**
   The experiment should be based on prior animal studies and a sound understanding of the disease or problem being studied, to justify the research.
4. **Avoid Unnecessary Suffering**
   The experiment should be conducted to avoid all unnecessary physical and mental suffering and injury.
5. **No Experiment if Death or Disability Is Expected**
   No experiment should be conducted where there is an a priori reason to believe death or disabling injury will occur—unless the physicians also serve as subjects.
6. **Risk Must Be Proportional to Benefit**
   The degree of risk taken should never exceed the humanitarian importance of the problem the experiment seeks to solve.
7. **Proper Preparations and Facilities**
   Adequate preparations must be made and proper facilities provided to protect subjects against even remote possibilities of harm.
8. **Only Qualified Personnel**
   The experiment should be conducted only by scientifically qualified persons. The highest degree of skill and care must be used throughout.
9. **Subject's Right to Withdraw**
   The human subject must be free to stop participation at any point if they feel physically or mentally unable to continue.
10. **Researcher Must Be Ready to Terminate**
    The scientist must be prepared to end the experiment at any stage if continuing it is likely to result in injury, disability, or death to the subject (Fig. 20.2).

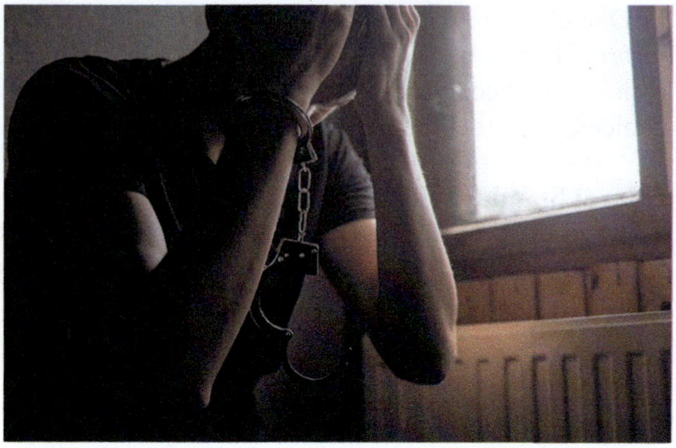

Fig. 20.2 The agony of prison

The Belmont Report [2]

The Belmont Report is a foundational document in research ethics in the United States. It was published in 1979 by the National Commission for the Protection of Human Subjects of Biomedical and Behavioral Research. Report emerged in response to a series of unethical research practices and scandals, most notably the Tuskegee syphilis study.

The Tuskegee syphilis study carried out between 1932 and 1972 was an infamous study of African American men with syphilis who were deliberately left untreated so researchers could study the natural progression of the disease even after effective treatment became available. The participants were not informed of their diagnosis or treatment options. Following a public outrage over the Tuskegee study and other unethical research practices Congress passed act establishing the National Commission for the participation of human subjects. The result of this Commission was the Belmont report which was officially published in April 1979.

The Belmont Report identifies three core ethical principles:

1. **Respect for Persons**
   - Individuals should be treated as autonomous agents.
   - People with diminished autonomy (e.g., children, individuals with cognitive impairment) are entitled to additional protections.
   - This principle underlies the need for **informed consent**.
2. **Beneficence**
   - Researchers must maximize possible benefits and minimize potential harms.
   - This includes conducting a **risk-benefit analysis** before and during the research.
3. **Justice**
   - The benefits and burdens of research should be distributed fairly.
   - This means ensuring equitable selection of subjects and avoiding exploitation of vulnerable populations.

Distinguishing Between Research and Practice

In research ethics, it's essential to understand the difference between **biomedical and behavioral research** and the **practice of accepted therapy.** This distinction is critical when determining which activities require ethical review to protect human subjects.

Research vs. Practice: Why the Confusion?

Research and clinical practice can often look similar—sometimes they happen at the same time. That overlap can cause confusion, especially since the word **"experimental"** is often used loosely. Just because a medical procedure is new or unfamiliar doesn't necessarily mean it qualifies as research.

What Is "Practice"?

The term **practice** refers to interventions designed **solely to enhance the well-being of an individual patient**, with a **reasonable expectation of success**. This includes:

- Diagnosis
- Preventive treatment
- Therapeutic procedures

In short, the goal of practice is to help **a specific person**, not to contribute to general knowledge.

What Is "Research"?

By contrast, **research** is a structured activity designed to:

- **Test a hypothesis**
- **Draw generalizable conclusions**
- **Contribute to broader scientific knowledge**

Research is typically guided by a formal **protocol**—a detailed plan that outlines objectives and procedures.

Even if a treatment is labeled "experimental," that alone doesn't make it research. However, **radically new procedures** should undergo formal research **early on** to assess their safety and effectiveness.

When Research and Practice Overlap

There are cases where research and practice happen **simultaneously**, such as when a new therapy is being evaluated during clinical care. In these cases, **research ethics guidelines still apply.**

Ethical Principles Governing Research

When human subjects are involved, three core ethical principles must guide research, as outlined in the **Belmont Report:**

Respect for Persons

This principle has two key components:

- **Acknowledging autonomy**:
  Individuals capable of making their own decisions should be allowed to do so. Respecting autonomy means:
  - Providing all necessary information for informed decision-making
  - Honoring individuals' choices unless those choices harm others
  - Not manipulating or coercing participants
- **Protecting those with diminished autonomy**:
  Some people—like children, those with cognitive impairments, or those facing severe constraints—cannot fully exercise self-determination. They require **additional protections.**
  The level of protection should match the level of risk and the individual's capacity to understand or consent. Importantly, a person's autonomy status should be **regularly reassessed**, as it can change over time or with context.

Beneficence

"Do no harm" is a long-standing principle of medical ethics. But **beneficence** goes further—it's not just about avoiding harm but also about actively promoting the **well-being of participants**.

In research ethics, beneficence means:

1. **Do not harm**
2. **Maximize possible benefits**
3. **Minimize possible harms**

Although the term is often associated with kindness or charity, in the Belmont Report, **beneficence is treated as a duty**, not an option.

Balancing Risk and Benefit

Some level of risk may be necessary in order to discover treatments or advance science. But the key ethical challenge is to determine: when it's justifiable to expose participants to risk and when the potential benefits do **not** outweigh the harm. Even when seeking valuable knowledge, researchers must prioritize safety and justify the design of their studies.

Who Holds This Obligation?

- **Researchers** must design studies that minimize risk and enhance benefit.
- **Institutions** must review and monitor research for ethical compliance.
- **Society** has a responsibility to support safe, ethical research that benefits all.

Justice

Who should benefit from research—and who bears its risks?

Justice in research is about **fairness in distribution**: No person or group should bear an unfair share of the burdens and no one should be denied benefits without valid reason. An **injustice** occurs when people are: excluded unfairly from potential benefits and selected for risky research merely due to vulnerability or ease of access.

Informed Consent

Respect for persons requires that individuals decide what happens to them. **Informed consent** is how this respect is applied in practice.

To be valid, informed consent must include:

1. **Information**
2. **Comprehension**
3. **Voluntariness**

Information

Subjects must be told:

- The purpose of the research
- The procedures involved
- Risks and possible benefits
- Alternatives (if any)
- Their right to ask questions and withdraw at any time

In some cases, full disclosure isn't possible before the study (e.g., in behavioral studies with incomplete information). In such cases:

- Deception must be necessary,
- Risk must remain minimal, and
- Debriefing must occur afterward.

Information about risk should never be withheld to gain cooperation.

Comprehension

The way information is presented is as important as the content. Factors like language, literacy, and cultural understanding affect a person's ability to give truly informed consent.

Researchers must:

- Ensure the participant understands the information
- Adapt communication to the participant's ability
- Reassess understanding, especially when risk is high

For individuals with limited capacity (children, cognitively impaired, etc.), extra safeguards—like seeking permission from guardians—must be in place.

Voluntariness

Consent must be given freely, without:

- Coercion (threats or pressure)
- Undue influence (excessive or inappropriate rewards)

Special care is needed when participants are in dependent or vulnerable positions—such as patients, prisoners, or students—where refusal might feel difficult or risky.

Risk-Benefit Assessment

Beneficence demands that risks be justified by the potential benefits, either to the individual participant or to society through gained knowledge.

What Counts as Risk or Benefit?

- **Risk** = the chance and severity of harm (physical, psychological, social, legal, or economic)
- **Benefit** = a valued positive outcome, usually related to health or welfare

Not all harms are obvious or immediate. Ethical review must weigh:

- Risks to the individual
- Risks to the individual's family or community
- Societal risks (e.g., stigmatization, misuse of data)

Researchers, IRBs, and funders must ensure that:

- Risks are minimized
- Benefits are maximized
- Alternatives are considered
- High-risk studies are carefully justified

Final Ethical Requirements

In applying all three Belmont principles—respect for persons, beneficence, and justice—researchers must meet these core ethical requirements:

Informed Consent

1. **Risk-benefit analysis**
2. **Fair selection of subjects**

These requirements form the ethical backbone of modern human subjects research.

Comprehension: More Than Just Giving Information

Ensuring that participants understand what they're agreeing to is just as important as providing them with the facts. If information is presented too quickly, disorganized, or without time for questions, participants may not fully grasp the risks or their rights. That's why comprehension must be tailored to each person's abili**ties**—accounting for factors like age, maturity, language skills, and cognitive capacity. Researchers have a duty to make sure participants:

- Understand what participation involves
- Are given time and clarity to consider their choices
- Are not misled or overwhelmed by technical jargon

In high-risk studies, extra care should be taken—sometimes even using quizzes or summaries to verify understanding. What About those with Limited Capacity? Participants like young children, cognitively impaired individuals, or people with serious illnesses may not be fully capable of informed consent. Still, they deserve:

As much choice as possible; protection from harm; and representation by someone who understands and acts in their best interest. Even if they can't legally consent, their objections should be respected unless the research provides life-saving care unavailable elsewhere. Guardians or representatives should also be allowed to monitor the research and withdraw the participant if necessary.

Voluntariness: Consent Must Be Freely Given

Consent is only valid if it's given voluntarily, without pressure, manipulation, or exploitation. Coercion happens when someone is threatened into saying yes. Undue influence involves excessive or inappropriate rewards that make it hard to say no—especially dangerous when participants are vulnerable or desperate.

For example:

- A doctor suggesting participation while controlling a patient's care may pressure them unfairly.
- Promising large rewards to someone in poverty may be ethically questionable.

Researchers must ensure that people say yes because they truly want to, not because they feel they have to.

Risk & Benefit Assessment: Balancing Safety with Scientific Value

Every research project must be carefully evaluated to make sure **that the potential benefits outweigh the risks.**

This process involves:

- **Identifying possible harms**—physical, psychological, social, legal, or economic
- **Estimating the likelihood and severity** of those harms
- **Weighing them against the expected benefits**—to the participant and to society

What's Considered a Risk or Benefit?

- **Risk** = the chance and severity of possible harm
- **Benefit** = a valuable outcome, like improved health or knowledge
- Risk/benefit analysis isn't about precise math—it's about making informed, ethical judgments using all available information

When considering harm include:

- Physical pain or injury
- Psychological distress
- Stigmatization
- Loss of privacy or legal rights

Review boards (IRBs) have a responsibility to ensure:

1. Brutal or inhumane research is never allowed.
2. Risks are minimized as much as possible
3. Research using high-risk methods must show strong justification.
4. Vulnerable groups are only included when necessary.
5. All risks and benefits are clearly explained in the consent process.

Subject Selection: Ensuring Fairness and Equity

Ethical research must also be fair in who it involves. This is where the principle of justice comes in.

There are two levels:

- **Individual justice**—Don't offer beneficial research only to favored groups or target disadvantaged ones for high-risk studies
- **Social justice**—Avoid placing the burdens of research on those already burdened (e.g., institutionalized people, prisoners, the poor)

Avoiding Exploitation

Historically, certain groups—like racial minorities, low-income populations, and the sick—have been overused in research because they're: readily available, less able to say no, and are dependent on the institutions or services provided.

To prevent exploitation:

- Vulnerable groups must be involved only when ethically justified.
- Adults should be considered before children, and those with fewer burdens before those with more.
- Publicly funded research should not benefit only the wealthy while using the disadvantaged as test subjects.

Summary: Ethical Safeguards in Research

The principles of the **Belmont Report** guide how we treat human subjects in research. Here's how they apply:

Principle	Ethical Application
Respect for persons	Informed consent & honoring autonomy
Beneficence	Minimize harm, maximize benefit
Justice	Fair selection & distribution of burdens

By upholding these principles, researchers, institutions, and society help ensure that science serves humanity—without exploiting it.

References

1. McCarthy K. The Nuremberg Code: 75th anniversary commemorative edition. Austin: Brasscheck Press; 2022.
2. The Belmont report: ethical principles and guidelines for the protection of human subjects of research. United States National Commission for the protection of human subjects of biomedical and behavioral research. Reprinted from the collection of the University of Michigan library.

Finding the Joy and Happiness

21

Not what we have, but what we enjoy constitutes our abundance. (Epicurus)

The Pure Joy of Medicine

There's a unique happiness that comes from practicing medicine [1]. It's the joy of connecting with patients, of helping them through their struggles, and the satisfaction that comes from solving complex medical puzzles. Whether it's the thrill of making a life-saving diagnosis, the joy of performing a successful surgery, or simply the camaraderie of working with bright, compassionate colleagues, medicine offers profound emotional and intellectual rewards. In medicine, we don't just heal bodies—we touch lives, build relationships, and, most importantly, contribute to the well-being of others. It is spiritually fulfilling, emotionally satisfying, and intellectually exhilarating. Medicine can be a source of constant joy, offering a sense of purpose that transcends the inevitable challenges and hardships of the profession [2] (Fig. 21.1).

B. Silverman, *The Power of Bedside Manners in Patient Care*,
https://doi.org/10.1007/978-3-032-10496-0_21

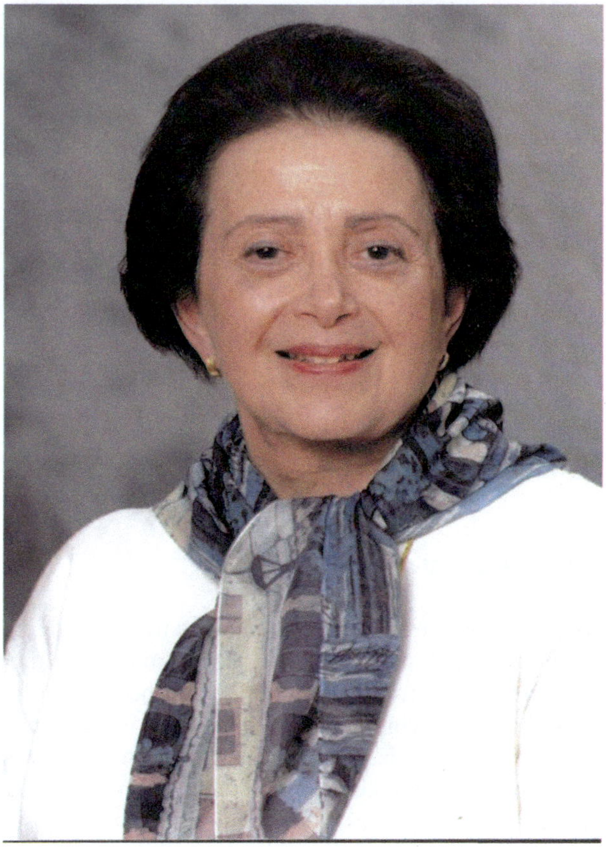

Fig. 21.1 Nanette K. Wenger. (Photo courtesy of Dr. Wenger)A giant in the field of cardiology whose groundbreaking research changed a major paradigm in medicine: the assumption that heart disease affects only men. Her enthusiasm on ward and in the clinics has inspired generations of young physicians

Sustaining Your Passion: Keeping the Flame Alive

As you journey through your medical career, it's essential to nurture the passion that brought you to medicine in the first place. At times, the pressures of patient care, the long hours, and the emotional toll of the work can cause that passion to wane. But by staying connected to the parts of the profession you love, you can rekindle your sense of purpose.

One way to maintain your enthusiasm is through community involvement. Whether it's volunteering at public hospitals, joining professional societies, or teaching medical students and the wider community, these activities allow you to engage with your profession in new and rewarding ways. Teaching, in particular, can offer a refreshing break from routine clinical work, allowing you to interact with students and trainees, and to share your knowledge and passion with the next generation of doctors.

Likewise, clinical research offers a stimulating and deeply gratifying avenue to explore. Medicine is constantly evolving, and research begins with observations made at the bedside. As a trained observer, you are uniquely positioned to contribute to the advancement of medical knowledge. Writing papers, serving as an editor for journals, or contributing to online resources can also offer intellectually satisfying ways to remain engaged with your field while making a lasting impact.

The Elements of a Successful Career

A fulfilling career in medicine requires more than just technical skill—it requires perseverance, commitment, and an ongoing pursuit of learning. Success in medicine comes not from avoiding challenges but from confronting them with a clear sense of purpose. You must continuously assess what you enjoy most about your work and focus on those aspects. Whether it's patient care, research, teaching, or leadership, identifying your core interests can help you find lasting satisfaction.

However, it's important to acknowledge that medicine is a demanding field, and at times, you may feel disconnected from the joy that once motivated you. When this happens, take time for self-reflection. Consider what truly drives you and seek out those aspects of medicine that reignite your passion. You may find that, even in the midst of adversity, the rewards of medicine are more than enough to sustain you.

Conclusion

The joy of medicine is multifaceted and enduring. Whether through direct patient care, teaching, research, or service to your community, medicine offers unique opportunities to experience personal fulfillment. The key to a successful, joyful career is to remain connected to the aspects of the profession that resonate most deeply with you, and to embrace every opportunity to learn, grow, and contribute.

In the words of Dr. Michael DeBakey: "Medicine is not just about solving problems; it's about making a difference." And it's this difference that brings joy—not only to the lives of the patients you care for but to your own life as well [3].

References

1. Servint JR. Cultivating the joy of medicine: a focus on intrinsic factors and the meaning of our work. Curr Probl Pediatr Adoles Health Care. 2019. PMID:31582295.
2. Thomas H. Where the joy comes from: a qualitative exploration of deep GP-patient relationships. BMC Prim Care. 2023. PMD 38087212.
3. Manning PR, DeBakey L, editors. Medicine: preserving the passion in the 21st century. New York: Springer; 2004.

Index

B. Silverman, *The Power of Bedside Manners in Patient Care*,
https://doi.org/10.1007/978-3-032-10496-0

9783032104953